*Nursing the Neurological
and Neurotrauma Patient*

Nursing the Neurological and Neurotrauma Patient

MARIA J. KRUSE

Rowman & Allanheld
PUBLISHERS

ROWMAN & ALLANHELD

Published in the United States of America in 1986
by Rowman & Allanheld, Publishers
(a division of Littlefield, Adams & Company)
81 Adams Drive, Totowa, New Jersey 07512.

Copyright © 1986 by Maria J. Kruse

All rights reserved. No part of this publication may be reproduced, stored in a retrieval system, or transmitted in any form or by any means, electronic, mechanical, photocopying, recording, or otherwise, without the prior permission of the publisher.

Library of Congress Cataloging-in-Publication Data

Kruse, Maria J.
   Nursing the neurological and neurotrauma patient.

   Bibliography: p. 105
   Includes index.
   1. Neurological nursing.   2. Nervous system—
Wounds and injuries—Nursing.   I. Title.
[DNLM: 1. Nervous System—injuries—nurses' instruction.
2. Nervous System Diseases—nursing.   WY 160 K94n]
RC350.5.K78   1986   617'.48044   85-27837
ISBN 0-8476-7451-7
ISBN 0-8476-7457-6 (pbk.)

86 87 88 / 10 9 8 7 6 5 4 3 2 1

Printed in the United States of America

*This book is dedicated to all my former patients,
who have given me more insight into human understanding
and endurance than I could ever repay.
My sincerest thanks to all of them.*

CONTENTS

Illustrations — x

INTRODUCTION — 1

CHAPTER 1. THE CELLULAR STRUCTURE OF THE NERVOUS SYSTEM — 4
Types of Nerve Cells and Their Functions — 4
The Role of Hormones in Nerve Conduction — 11

CHAPTER 2. THE BRAIN — 12
Protective Structures of the Brain and Spinal Cord — 12
Anatomical Structure of the Brain — 14
   The Cerebral Cortex, 15 The Thalamus and Hypothalamus, 17 The Midbrain, 18 The Pons, 18 The Cerebellum, 18 Medulla Oblongata, 19

CHAPTER 3. THE SPINAL CORD AND CENTRAL NERVOUS SYSTEM FUNCTIONS — 21
Structure of the Spinal Cord — 21
   The Spinal Nerves, 22 Spinal Tap, 25
Sensory Neural Pathways — 27
Motor Neural Pathways — 29
The Reticular Activating System — 31
Reflexes — 32
   Knee Jerk or Patellar Reflex, 32 Ankle Jerk, 32 Babinski Reflex, 32 Corneal Reflex, 33 Abdominal Reflex, 33 Gag and Cough Reflex, 33 Swallowing or Palatal Reflex, 33
Autonomic Nervous System — 34
The Balancing Function of the Autonomic Nervous System — 35

CHAPTER 4. THE CRANIAL NERVES — 37
How to Test the Cranial Nerves — 37

CHAPTER 5. INTRACRANIAL PRESSURE — 46
Signs and Symptoms of Increased ICP — 50
Monitoring the Intracranial Pressure — 51

CHAPTER 6. ASSESSMENT OF THE NEUROLOGICAL PATIENT AND THE NURSE'S ROLE IN TREATMENT AND CARE — 53
Neurological Assessment — 53
Injuries to the Central Nervous System — 56
Evaluating the Level of Consciousness — 57
Monitoring and Treatment of the Unconscious Patient — 58
Supportive Treatment and Nursing Care — 61
The Convulsing Patient — 62

CHAPTER 7. HEAD INJURIES — 65
Open Head Injuries — 65
Closed Head Injuries — 67
Medical Management of Skull Fractures — 69

CHAPTER 8. SPINAL CORD INJURIES — 70
Types of Spinal Cord Lesions and Their Physiological Effects — 70
Evaluation and Management of Spinal Injuries — 74
Nursing Management of the Patient with Spinal Cord Injury or Lesions — 78
   Ventilation, Circulation, Elimination, and Assimilation, 78
   Intake and Output, 79 Medication, 79 Emotional Needs, 80

CHAPTER 9. ACUTE MEDICAL-NEUROLOGIC CONDITIONS — 82
Strokes and Hypertension — 82
Assessment and Management of Patients with Strokes — 84
Subarachnoid Hemorrhage — 86
Poliomyelitis — 87
Encephalitis — 88
Meningitis — 89
Tetanus (Lockjaw) — 90
Guillain-Barré Syndrome — 91
Myasthenia Gravis — 92

CHAPTER 10. NEUROLOGICAL DIAGNOSTIC STUDIES — 95

The Electroencephalogram (EEG) — 95
Echoencephalography — 96
Pneumoencephalography — 96
Spinal Tap or Lumbar Puncture — 97
Radiographic Studies — 97
Cerebral Angiography — 97
Ventriculography — 98
Myelography — 99
Brain Scanning with Radioisotopes — 100
Computer-Assisted Tomography — 101
Caloric Test for Vestibular Function — 102
Glucose Tolerance Test — 102
Iodine-Starch Sweat Test — 103

REFERENCES — 105

GLOSSARY OF TERMS — 109

APPENDICES — 119
Major Neurological Drugs — 119
Abbreviations — 127

INDEX — 129

ILLUSTRATIONS

FIGURES

1.1	Astrocyte I—Fibrous Astrocyte of the White Matter	6
1.2	Astrocyte II—Protoplasmic, Non-fibrous Astrocyte of the Gray Matter	6
1.3	Microglial Cell, with Processes Extending to Two Nerve Cells	7
1.4	Two Oligodendroglial Cells Near a Nerve Cell	7
1.5	Diagram of Neuron and Axon	9
2.1	Brain Coverings and Ventricles	13
2.2	Sagittal Section of the Brain	15
2.3	Major Areas of the Brain, Showing Specific Function of the Cerebral Cortex	16
3.1	Cross-section of Vertebra and Spinal Cord	21
3.2	Spinal Cord Levels	23
3.3	Cross-section of Spinal Cord, Showing Some of the Major Spinothalamic Tracts	24
3.4	Cross-section of Spinal Cord, Including Spinal Nerves as They Exit the Cord	24
5.1	Cycle of Progressive Neurological Deficit Resulting from Evolving Cerebral Edema	49
5.2	Neurological Assessment—Glasgow Coma Scale	52
8.1	Dermatomes—Front and Back Views	71

TABLE

4.1	The Cranial Nerves	38

INTRODUCTION

Volumes could be written on each of the topics touched upon in this text on neurological and neurotrauma nursing. The intention, however, has been to keep this book short, simple, and easy to read so that it may be used as a quick reference. Designed as an aid to all who render care to these patients, it is geared to both nursing students in their senior year and new graduates who have an interest in this branch of nursing and wish to prepare to work in the neurological or neurotrauma clinical areas. For Registered Nurses who are returning to nursing it may serve as a refresher, and for nurses in other clinical areas it will provide a brief but concise update to help them become more proficient in meeting the needs of the patient with neurological deficits—especially if they wish to work in acute care areas such as the intensive care unit or the emergency department. Intended to help the nurse become more familiar with or interested in caring for neurological and neurotrauma patients in the acute phase, this text is designed to dispel some of the fears and mysteries usually associated with neurotrauma nursing and, it is hoped, to enhance the knowledge of those already working in these clinical areas. Last, paramedics and emergency medical technicians—the first-line care providers of the neurotrauma victim in the field—should find the book useful, especially the sections on neurological assessment and the initial care of the spinal cord–injured patient.

The patient with neurological disorders challenges the observational powers and bedside skills of those who care for him—the physician, the nurse, the radiological technologist, the physical therapist, and so on. As in any other health care endeavor, careful observation and recording are important, but in this area even the slightest changes in neurological function are of paramount importance. The better we understand the symptoms of various neurological disorders, the more perceptive we will become in observation and the more accurate in interpreting changes and their implications. With this information, we are able to formulate and carry out a plan of action in caring for the patient with neurological deficits.

A good basic understanding of the body's nervous system is a prerequisite for care providers to enable them to render safe and effective care based on sound clinical principles. They must be familiar with the morphological aspects of the nervous system, its composition, its shape or form, and how it integrates with other body systems. They must know what makes it tick, so to speak, and what keeps it from optimal operation. They must be able to do a neurological assessment, know the accepted parameters for normal physiological and psychological functions, and be able to formulate a valid plan for the care of the patient with various neurological disorders or deficits. The scope of this text does not permit an in-depth review of the anatomy and physiology of the nervous system in a healthy individual. The focus will be on pathophysiological events, how they occur, and how to deal with them. It also includes a brief section on psychological changes that may occur whenever there are interruptions in the sensory and motor pathways. Therefore, throughout the text, the role of accurate observation and interpretation of symptoms is stressed.

The text includes a brief overview of the anatomy and physiology of the human nervous system, with stress placed on pathophysiological events and how to deal with them. The relevant anatomical structures are treated according to location and function. Included are cellular differentiation and its role within the system; the skull; the brain with its lobes and coverings; the ventricles; the spine with its vertebrae and their role; the spinal cord and its coverings; the cerebrospinal fluid (CSF), its role and composition; the cranial nerves, their location, origin, function, and how to test them; and the major reflexes.

It also includes a section on physical assessment of the neurological patient; the use of the Glasgow Coma Scale as an assessment tool; various laboratory, radiological, and specific neurological studies; the causes and effects of cerebral edema and signs and symptoms of increased intracranial pressure (ICP), and their clinical implications. Other topics include nursing management of the neurotrauma victim with head and/or spinal cord injuries; and the care of the unconscious patient, as well as the patient with seizures, cerebral vascular accident (CVA), subarachnoid hemorrhage (SAH), meningitis, myasthenia gravis crisis, tetanus, encephalitis, poliomyelitis, and Guillain-Barré Syndrome. The most commonly performed neurological diagnostic tests are described; a glossary of terms and a list of the most commonly used drugs in neurological and neurotrauma nursing are provided.

CHAPTER 1 | THE CELLULAR STRUCTURE OF THE NERVOUS SYSTEM

Integration and control of the body are maintained by the nervous system. Even the simplest activities require complicated actions within it, and unless all parts of the system are functioning effectively it is impossible to perform these actions. Let us look at the simple task of tying a shoelace. This would not be possible if the portion of the brain controlling this function or the nerves in the arms or hands were damaged. If only the nerves in the arms or hands were damaged, one would still be unable to tie the shoelace, even though the brain willed the arms and hands to do so. There must be uninterrupted communication between the nervous system and the rest of the body for it to function correctly; in fact, survival depends on it. If there is a disruption within the system or in its ability to communicate, sensory or motor dysfunctions will result.

Communication, in this context, refers to the nervous system's ability to receive and send messages—its ability to exchange information. The body has two communication devices: nerve impulses and chemicals, such as hormones. Since the intent of this text is to study the nervous system, chemicals will be discussed only when necessary for clarification of bodily functions as they relate to total body integration and control.

In reviewing the anatomical structures and functions of the human nervous system, we will begin with the types of cells that make up the system.

TYPES OF NERVE CELLS AND THEIR FUNCTIONS

There are two basic types of nerve cells, the *neuroglia* and the *neurons*. There are three different neuroglial cells identified histologically and classified according to their functions:

1. The star-shaped *astrocytes* (see Figures 1.1 and 1.2) with numerous processes that form a supporting network for the neurons (nerve cells) and attach them to the surrounding blood vessels by little "sucker feet."
2. The *microglial* cells (see Figure 1.3), which are very small and move freely about in the brain tissue and are phagocytic in their function if there is inflammation or tissue death.
3. The *oligodendroglial* cells, which have fewer processes (see Figure 1.4) than the other two types but are also interposed between the neurons and their blood vessels.

In short, neuroglial cells support, connect, and protect the neurons as well as play a role in formation of the myelin sheath of neurons in the brain and spinal cord. (These cells have clinical implications in tumor formation and its growth in the central nervous system.)

Neurons (nerve cells) are classified according to their structure and function:

1. The *sensory* (afferent) *neurons*, which transmit nerve impulses to the spinal cord or the brain.
2. The *motor* (efferent) *neurons*, which transmit impulses away from the spinal cord or the brain. They are limited to the central nervous system (CNS).

As stated earlier, neurons are classified not only by their functions but also by their structure:

1. *Multipolar neurons*, which have multiple processes coming off the cell body—several dentrites but only one axon. Most of the neurons in the brain and spinal cord fall into this class.
2. *Bipolar neurons*, which have two processes coming off the cell body—one dentrite and one axon. They are found in the retina of the eye and the spiral ganglion of the inner ear.
3. *Unipolar neurons*, which have only one process (an axon) coming off the cell body. Although these neurons are called unipolar they function as bipolar neurons. As the process (axon) leaves the cell body it splits into two processes for a brief distance, after which the two processes intertwine to become one again. The single process divides once again into two branches—a peripheral branch that functions as a dentrite, and a central branch that functions as an axon. Most

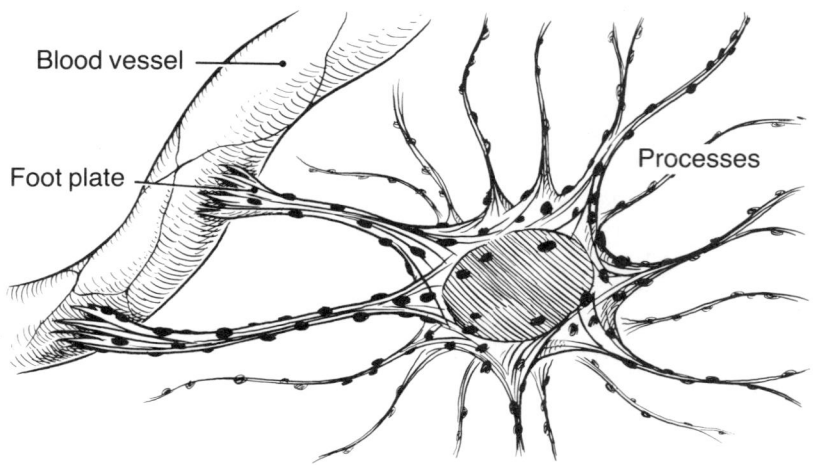

Figure 1.1. Astrocyte I—Fibrous astrocyte of the white matter, with foot plate against blood vessels and numerous processes serving as support for the neurons.

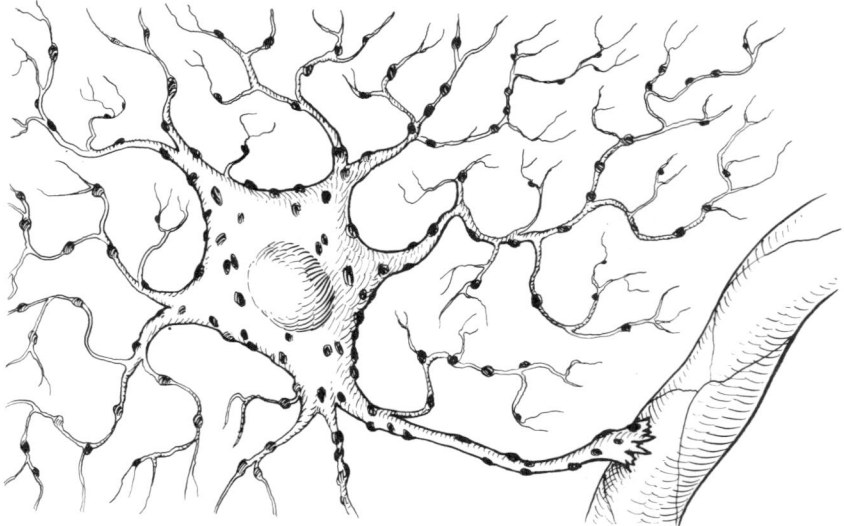

Figure 1.2. Astrocyte II—Protoplasmic, non-fibrous astrocyte of the gray matter.

The Cellular Structure of the Nervous System 7

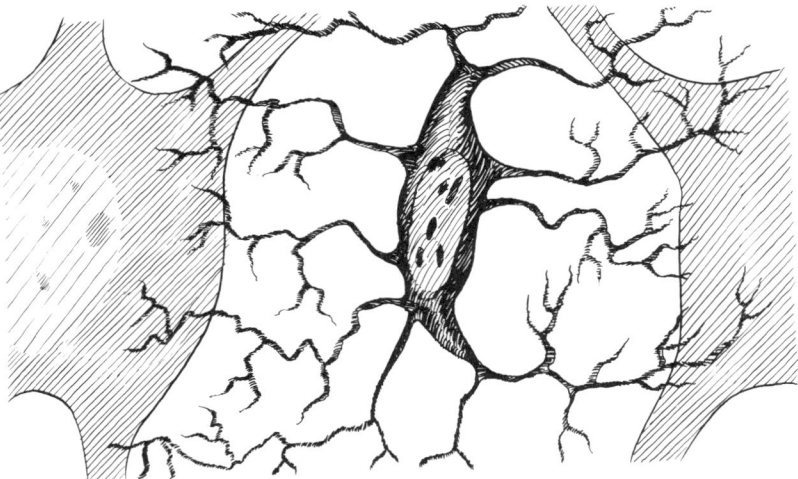

Figure 1.3. Microglial cell, with processes extending to two nerve cells.

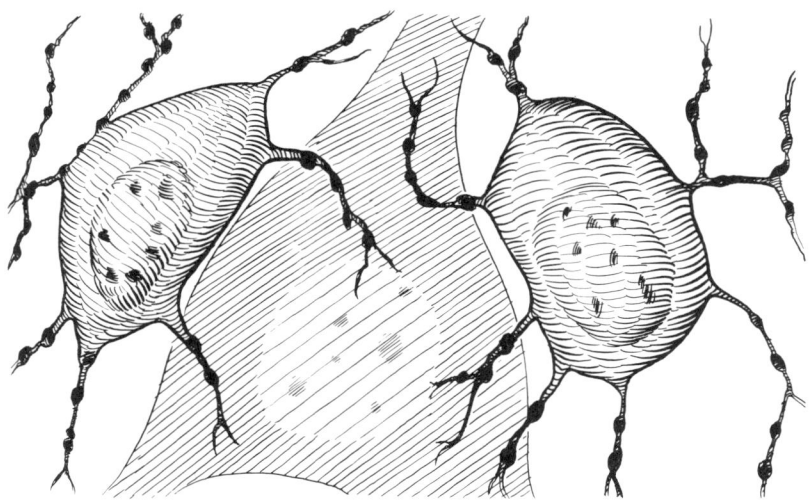

Figure 1.4. Two oligodendroglial cells near a nerve cell.

peripheral sensory neurons fall into this class or are unipolar.

The basic function of neurons is to respond to stimuli by transmitting nerve impulses. They provide the body with irritability and conductivity.

The structural elements characteristic of neurons (see Figure 1.5) are dendrites, axon, myelin sheath, neurilemma, neurofibrils, and nissl bodies. *Dendrite(s)* is the process or processes, depending on the neuron being bipolar or multipolar, that extend out from the main part of the nerve cell and serve to conduct impulses to the body of the neuron. Each dendrite branches out to form a network, so that it resembles a little tree. ("Dendrite" is derived from the Greek *dendron,* meaning "tree.") The distal (terminal) ends of the dendrites of sensory neurons are called the receptors because they receive the initial stimulus.

Axons are single processes that extend from the neuron cell body and conduct impulses away from it. A neuron has only one axon, but this may, and does at times, branch out into axon collaterals. The axons, which vary in length from a few inches to as long as three feet or more, can carry impulses great distances from the cell body. They also vary in diameter, which allows varying velocities in the transmission of impulses. (The larger the diameter of an axon, the greater the velocity of impulse transmission.)

The *myelin sheath,* a segmental membrane covering the nerve fiber (axon), is composed of a double layer of cells, a type of structure known as Schwann's cells. The Schwann's cell membrane has a high proportion of liquid (fat) to protein and serves as an electrical insulator. These cells act as satellites for the nerve fibers located along the peripheral nerves.

The *neurilemma* is a continuous sheath around the segmental myelin sheath. This is also composed of Schwann's cells. The neurilemma plays an essential role in peripheral nerve fiber regeneration. The brain and spinal cord fibers do not contain neurilemma and are therefore not capable of regeneration. Once these fibers are destroyed by disease or injury the degeneration is permanent, resulting in neurological deficits with serious clinical implications.

Neurofibrils are the delicate interlacing of thread-like fibers

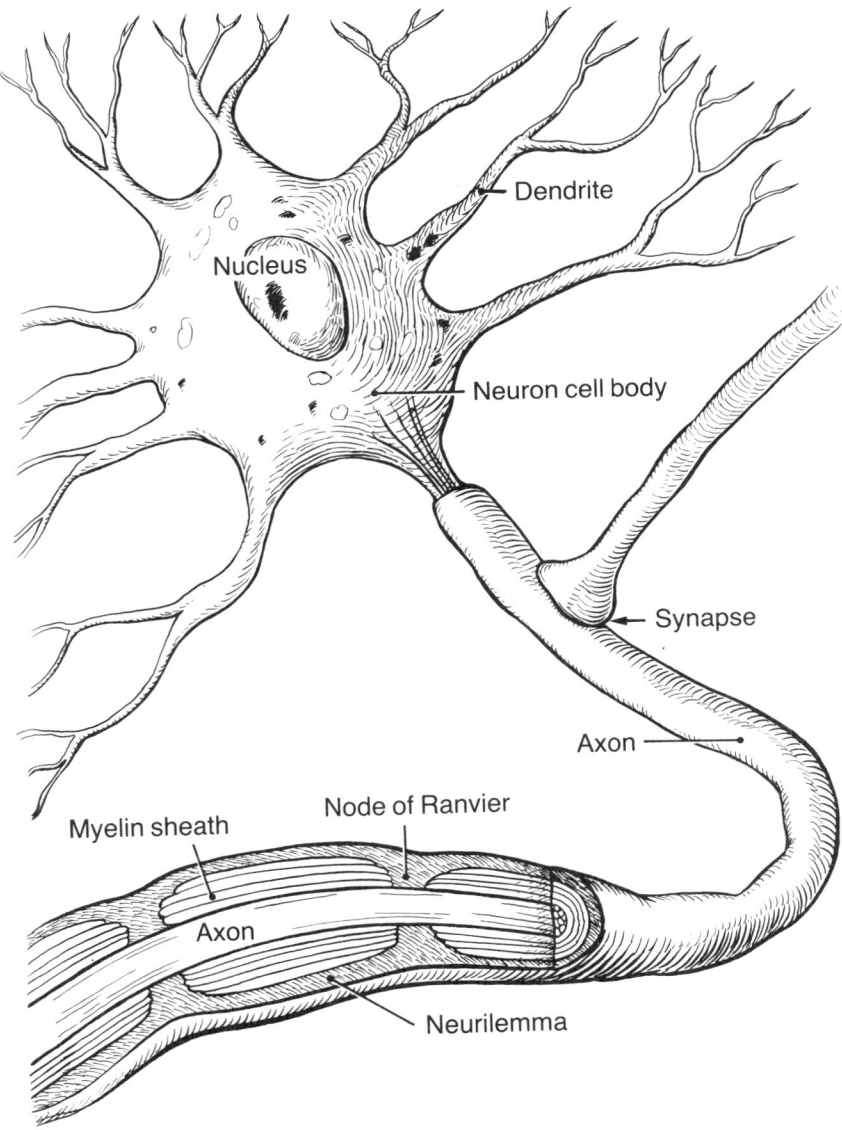

Figure 1.5. Diagram of neuron and axon.

coursing through the cytoplasm of the neuron (nerve cell body). They extend out to the dendrites and axon and are believed to be conducting elements.

Nissl bodies consist of groups of flat, membranous sacs and many RNA granules. They constitute the rough-surfaced vesicles of the endoplasmic reticulum of the neurons. These vesicles are minute sacs containing liquid high in protein, and are believed to be protein synthesizers and protein-bound humoral transmitters within the neuron. In short, they are the neuron's internal protein synthesizers and protein transport system.

To repeat, the function of neurons is to transmit or conduct impulses, at times at the speed of lightning. They provide a means for both rapid control of individual structures and for integration of the activities of many different structures.

Conduction of an impulse begins normally when a *stimulus* acts on a *receptor*. (A stimulus is a change in the pre-existing condition of the organism's environment. It may be internal or external, as a change in temperature or pressure.) The receptors—distal ends of the dendrites of the sensory neurons—very rapidly conduct the impulse induced by the stimulus to the cell body and axon. Whether or not a stimulus initiates a response depends on the intensity or strength of the stimulus and the receptor's ability to receive it and conduct an impulse. Impulse conduction begins with the stimulation of the receptors and ends with a response by *effectors* (muscles or glands). The routes that these impulses travel between receptors and effectors are called the *neural pathways* or *reflex arcs*. The cells that make up these pathways or reflex arcs are composed of neurons, the body's specialists in conduction. These reflex arcs can range from a simple two-neuron structure to extremely complex pathways. The two-neuron arc is composed of a single sensory neuron, a motoneuron, and a synapse.

The *synapse* is a contact point between the end of an axon filament of one neuron and the dendrite of another neuron. The speed with which an impulse is conducted, depending on the diameter of the axon fibers, can range from 0.5 to 100 meters per second.

THE ROLE OF HORMONES IN NERVE CONDUCTION

Many axons terminate in little knobs called *synaptic knobs,* or *end feet,* or sometimes *end buttons.* Each synaptic knob contacts a dendrite or a cell body of another neuron—this constitutes a synapse. There is no actual physical contact between these two points, however. A minute space exists between them, about one-millionth of an inch, which is called the *synaptic cleft.* To transmit an impulse across this minute space at some of the synapses, *acetylcholine,* a hormone, is secreted (the other exitatory transmitters are not known). *Cholinesterase,* the inhibitor of acetylcholine, is secreted within seconds and terminates the synaptic conduction.

Neuromuscular junctions are contact points (places) between a motoneuron's axon terminals and a muscle cell's membrane. Axons of motoneurons release acetylcholine at their junction with skeletal muscle cells. This initiates impulse conduction along the muscle cell membrane, and contraction follows almost immediately.

CHAPTER 2 | THE BRAIN

After a brief overview of the basic or cellular structure of the central nervous system, we next consider its organ structure. The organs of the central nervous system include the brain, spinal cord, nerves, and ganglia. The two main components are the brain and spinal cord; both these organs are very delicate and vital to survival. They are provided with three protective structures: bone, the meninges, and cerebrospinal fluid (for visual details see Figure 2.1).

PROTECTIVE STRUCTURES OF THE BRAIN AND SPINAL CORD

The outermost protection comes from the bone of the cranium for the brain and the vertebral column for the spinal cord. In addition to these bony protections, the brain and the spinal cord are covered by a tough, three-layered membrane known as the *meninges*. The three layers of the meninges are: the *dura mater*, which consists of a strong fibrous tissue that serves as the outer layer of the meninges and the inner lining of the cranial vault; *arachnoid membrane*, the delicate, cobweb-like middle layer; and the *pia mater*, a transparent layer of membrane containing the blood vessels, which adheres to the outer surface of the brain and spinal cord. A brief mention should be made here of the three extentions of the dura mater. The first is the *falx cerebri*, which extends downward into the longitudinal fissure to form a sort of partition between the left and right cerebral hemispheres of the brain. The second extension is the *falx cerebelli*, which separates the two cerebellar hemispheres. The third is the *tentorium cerebelli*, forming a tent-like covering over the cerebellum—hence its name. Between the dura mater and the arachnoid membrane is a small

The Brain

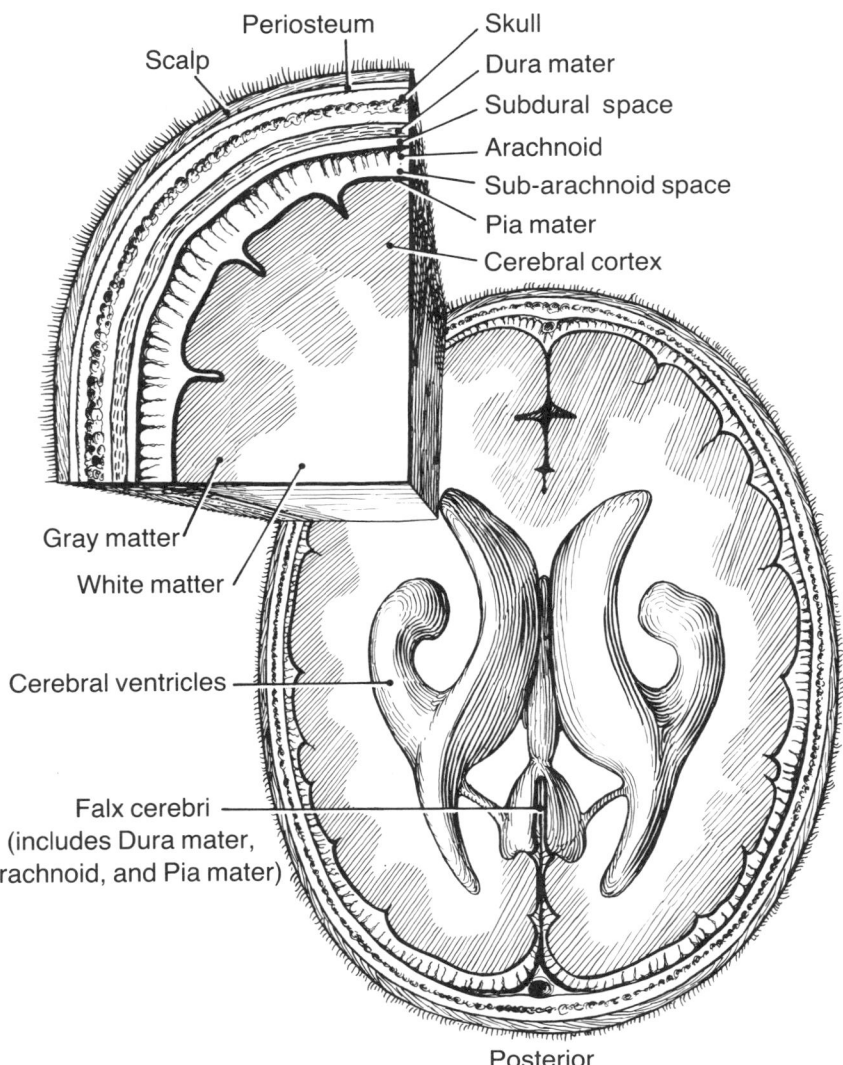

Figure 2.1. Brain coverings and ventricles, viewed from above.

space called the *subdural space*, and between the arachnoid membrane and pia mater is another small space called the *subarachnoid space*. The latter contains *cerebrospinal fluid* (CSF) to cushion the brain and the spinal cord from jarring injuries. In addition to protection afforded by the subarachnoid space in the brain and spinal cord, there are ventricles in the brain—four in all—as well as aqueducts and the central or spinal canal in the cord for further protection. The cerebrospinal fluid is clear (if not, there are significant clinical implications, which will be discussed later) and is formed primarily by filtration out of the blood by networks of capillaries.

ANATOMICAL STRUCTURE OF THE BRAIN

The brain and spinal cord make up the central nervous system, and the nerves and ganglia make up the peripheral nervous system. The following extremely brief review of the anatomical composition of the brain is intended to aid recall so that the text can be more easily understood.

To obtain a meaningful view of the brain, it is necessary to examine the structure of its parts according to the function that they perform. This approach aids in the interpretation of pathophysiological events and in identifying the part of the nervous system that is injured or diseased. The brain is one of the largest organs in the human adult. It weighs about three pounds. It is generally smaller in women than in men and smaller in older persons than in younger persons. The brain has three major divisions: the *forebrain* or *cerebrum* and two parts of the *diencephalon*—the *thalamus* and the *hypothalamus*. The cerebrum is divided into two halves, known as *hemispheres*. Each hemisphere is further subdivided into five lobes, four of which are named for the bone lying over them—that is, parietal, frontal, temporal, and occipital. The Island of Reil is the only lobe not named for the overlying bone.

Each hemisphere is composed of three parts: the *cerebral cortex*, the *tracts*, and the *basal ganglia* or *cerebral nuclei*, which is the more common term. (An area of gray matter is referred to as nucleus rather than basal ganglia, but a cluster of neuron cell bodies and

The Brain

dendrites located outside the brain and spinal cord are always referred to as basal ganglia.) The clusters of neuron cell bodies and dendrites in the brain resemble little sausages linked together, giving the cerebral cortex its characteristic convoluted appearance. The peaks and depths of this convolution can be measured by performing an electroencephalogram (EEG), a diagnostic procedure measuring the brain surface's electrical activity. If there is an interruption in these convolutions it is expressed by very spiked or flat waves on the EEG, and the person will have uncontrolled muscular activity known as seizures. The cerebral *tracts* are situated interiorly to the cortex and are composed of a great number of axons (nerve fibers). The cerebral tract's name reflects the two parts it connects—the first part where the axon originates and the second where it terminates—the corticospinal tract. There are both sensory and motor tracts.

The Cerebral Cortex

The largest part of the brain is the cerebral cortex (see Figures 2.2 and 2.3). Performing all mental functions, it is considered to be the intelligence center, and it controls many essential motor,

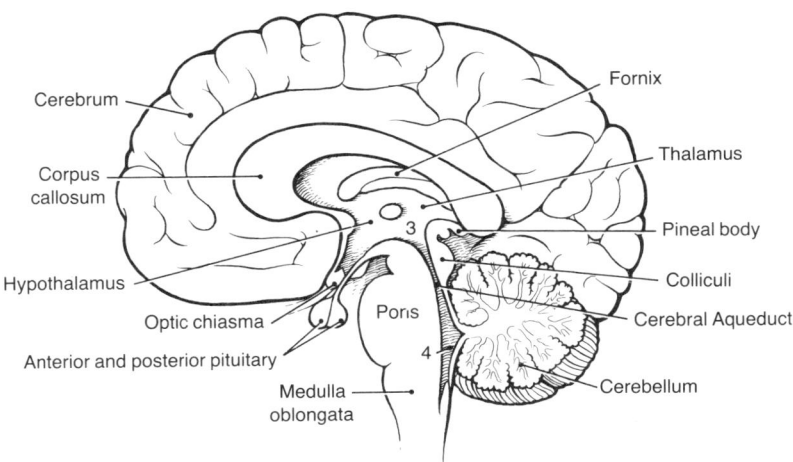

Figure 2.2. Sagital section of the brain.

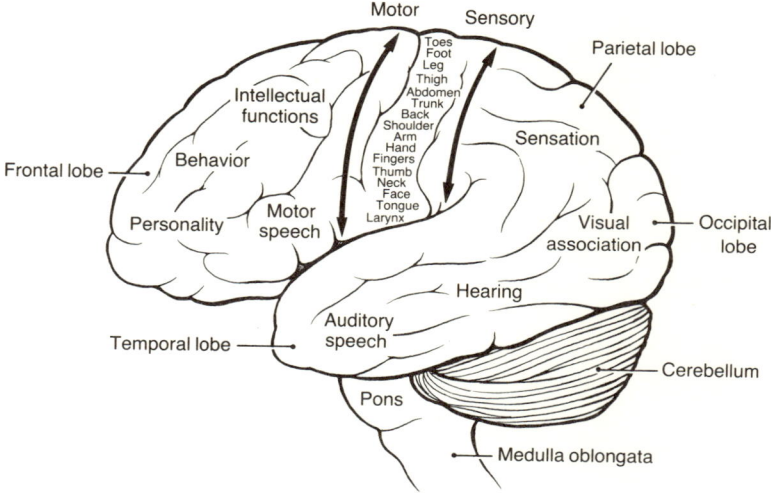

Figure 2.3. Major areas of the brain, showing the specific functions of the cerebral cortex (sensory and motor components).

sensory, and visceral functions as well. Blushing with embarrassment or turning pale with fear are examples of visceral change; they are caused by constriction and dilation of facial blood vessels controlled by the cerebral cortex. The frontal and temporal lobes are believed to be responsible for memory and emotions. If injury or disease occurs in these areas the effects on recall and emotional expression are revealed in deviation in personality traits and behavior.

Parts of the temporal lobe and the occipital lobe are responsible for our special senses—hearing, smelling, and vision. If there are impairments in these senses, the neurological disturbances are occurring in the above two areas. Speech difficulties or different types of aphasia, on the other hand, are related to the language centers of the cortex. There are three: the frontal, parietal, and temporal—the motor speech area being in the frontal lobe. If a lesion occurs here, the person will be unable to express himself—he will have expressive aphasia, although he is capable of speech.

The Thalamus and Hypothalamus

These two parts of the brain, which lie between the cortex and midbrain, are composed of gray matter and extend to the lateral wall of the third ventricle. Here the axons of the spinothalamic tracts terminate and synapse with neurons whose axons extend in the thalamocortical tracts to the general sensory area of the cerebral cortex. Thus, these nuclei serve as relay stations for the sensory impulses. Their function is the conscious recognition of crude pain, touch, and temperature. They also relay the special senses, with the exception of smell. In part, they are responsible for emotions, the arousal or alerting mechanism, and the production of complex reflex movements.

The hypothalamus is the link between the psyche (mind) and the soma (body). It links the nervous system to the endocrine system and controls the primary drives—eating, drinking, and mating. Referred to as the higher autonomic center, it sends impulses to the lower autonomic centers. Its tracts extend to the parasympathetic and sympathetic centers in the brainstem and spinal cord. By controlling the amount of hormone the posterior pituitary secretes, the hypothalamus maintains the body's water balance and many other cellular functions of the body. For its minute size, about one quarter of an ounce, it is a mighty giant functionally. Among its functions is the control of the body's temperature. If a lesion occurs in the hypothalamus, the body's temperature will rise to lethal heights and very little, if anything, can be done clinically for the patient.

A lesion within the nervous system is not simply an overgrowth of cells, such as a tumor, but an interruption in nerve conduction that can result from injury or other destruction of the system's integrity. Central nervous system lesions may result from a broken blood vessel in the brain (a CVA), from displaced vertebral fractures, or cell death from cerebral infarcts (like a myocardial infarction, due to the lack of adequate blood supply). These are but a few of the causes that lead to the interruption of normal neurological functions.

The Midbrain

The midbrain lies below the inferior surface of the cerebrum and above the pons. It consists mostly of white matter. The midbrain is a connecting tract between the forebrain and hindbrain, and the nuclei of the third, fourth, and fifth cranial nerves are located deep within it. It also contains some of the auditory and visual reflex nuclei—control of pupillary reaction is located here.

The Pons

Above the medulla lies the pons, which is composed of white matter and very few nuclei. The reticular formation extends into the pons from the medulla. One of the important reticular areas in the pons is the *pneumotaxic center*, which controls respiration. Nuclei from the fifth to the eighth cranial nerves lie in the upper part of the pons.

The Cerebellum

The cerebellum, the second largest part of the brain, is located below the posterior portion of the cerebrum, separated from it by a transverse fissure. They share some characteristics; the exterior of the cerebellum is also composed of gray matter and its interior of white matter, although there is proportionately less gray matter in the cerebellum. The vascular arrangement is much the same, and the cerebellar surface, or gray matter, is grooved with little sausage-like, convoluted formations. The convolutions, however, are less prominent—shallower—than those of the cerebrum. The internal white matter of the cerebellum is composed of some long but mainly short tracts. The short association tracts connect the cerebellar cortex with nuclei located in the interior of the cerebellum. The longer tracts connect the cerebellum with other parts of the brain and spinal cord. These tracts enter or leave the cerebellum by way of its three pairs of *peduncles* (a large bundle of nerve fibers): the interior, composed chiefly of tracts into the cerebellum from the medulla and spinal cord; the middle, composed almost entirely of tracts into the cerebellum from the pons; and the superior, tracts principally composed of dentate nuclei connecting the cerebellum with motor areas of the cerebral cortex. The impulses travel both ways via these tracts between their connecting points.

The three general functions of the cerebellum are to coordinate fine muscle motor movement within the cerebral cortex to produce motor coordination, to maintain muscular control or equilibrium and control of posture, and to make movements smooth instead of jerky, steady instead of trembling. If there is a lesion in the cerebellum, there will be asynergia, hypotonia, tremors, and disturbances in gait and equilibrium. One of the tests that is used in evaluation of cerebellar integrity is the finger-to-nose test. The staggering gait is another indication of cerebellar lesion. Cerebellar lesions do not cause paralysis; if it occurs its origin is in another part of the brain or spinal cord.

Medulla Oblongata

The medulla, which is also referred to as the bulb, brainstem, or vital center of the brain, is the extension of the spinal cord that passes through the *foramen magnum*, the large opening in the occipital lobe of the cranium. Located just above the foramen magnum at the base of the skull, it is composed mainly of white matter with projection tracts (gray matter) and reticular formation. The reticular formation is the interlacement of white and gray matter, present in the spinal cord, the brainstem, and the diencephalon of the brain. The nuclei in the reticular formation within the medulla oblongata are responsible for the control of respiration and vasomotor activities—the heart and blood vessels.

The medulla oblongata is the most vital part of the entire brain—so vital in fact, that injury or disease of the medulla often proves fatal. Blows to the base of the skull and bulbar poliomyelitis are examples of disordered states that can cause death if they interrupt impulse conduction in the vital centers of the brainstem. If a patient is presented in the emergency department or the ICU with a possible basilar skull fracture (an orbital blowout or stellate-type fracture creating an access to the brain) the nurse is never to suction this patient nasally (via the nares), as the suction catheter may go upward and enter through the opening created by the fractured bones and kill the patient. This type of patient is always suctioned through the mouth until the X-rays establish a firm diagnosis, or rule out basilar skull fracture. The medulla houses, in addition to the vital centers, two prominent nuclei—the *nucleus gracilis* and the *nucleus cuneatus*. These two nuclei are afferent fibers extending from the posterior white columns of the spinal cord synapse with neurons whose axons extend to the thalamus and cerebellum. The medulla also houses the *pyramids*—two bulges of white matter located on the anterior surface of the medulla formed by fibers of the pyramidal projection tracts—and the *olive*, which is an oval projection also located on each side of the anterior surface of the medulla. Fibers from these nuclei run through the interior cerebellar peduncles (also called *restiform bodies*) into the cerebellum. This provides connection between the cerebellum and the body.

Nuclei of the ninth through the twelfth cranial nerves are located in the medulla. The medulla thus houses a number of non-vital reflex centers as well as the vital centers of the body. The non-vital reflexes include the centers for vomiting, coughing, sneezing, hiccoughing, and swallowing, among others. All projection tracts between the spinal cord and brain pass through the medulla, which means that the medulla functions in a great many sensory as well as motor control mechanisms. The fibers of the corticospinal tracts cross over (decussate) from one side to the other in the pyramids of the medulla. This anatomical arrangement explains why one side of the brain is said to control the other side of the body (contralateral control). For instance, if the patient is paralyzed on the right side of his body, the lesion (disease) is affecting the left side of the brain; or if the patient's left pupil is dilated, the cerebral bleeding or edema is pressing on the right side of the occipital area of the cerebral cortex, where the nerve fibers of vision control are housed.

Following this brief review of the basic structures of the brain and some of its functions, we will consider the spinal cord, the other major organ of the central nervous system.

CHAPTER 3 | THE SPINAL CORD AND CENTRAL NERVOUS SYSTEM FUNCTIONS

STRUCTURE OF THE SPINAL CORD

Like the brain, the spinal cord has its three-way protection (see Figures 2.1 and 3.1) which is comprised of the outer bony protection (the vertebral column), the meninges, and the cerebrospinal fluid. The vertebral column includes eight cervical, twelve thoracic, and five lumbar vertebrae, the sacrum, and the coccyx. The latter two are a fusion of several vertebrae—five and four, respectively. In the average human adult body the length of the

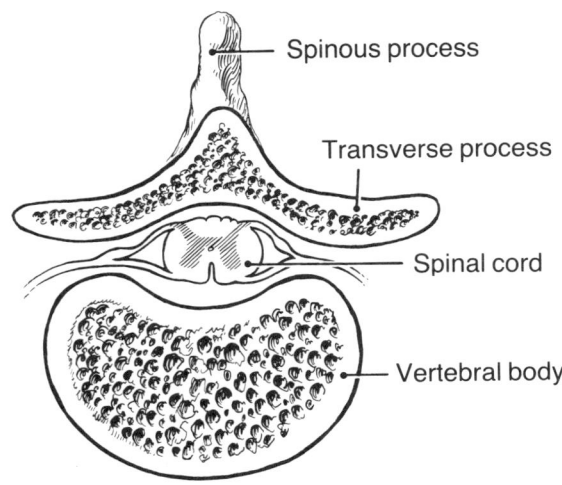

Figure 3.1. Cross-section of vertebra and spinal cord (through body of vertebra).

spinal cord is seventeen to eighteen inches. It lies within the spinal cavity and extends from the foramen magnum to the lower border of the first lumbar vertebra.

Although the spinal cord extends only to the first lumbar vertebra, its covering (meninges) continues into the sacral area, and the pia mater (inner covering) forms slender filaments known as the *filum terminale*. The filum terminale blends with the dura mater (outer covering of the spinal cord) at the third sacral vertebra to form a fibrous cord that disappears into the periosteum of the coccyx (see Figure 3.2). The spinal cord itself is an oval-shaped cylinder that tapers as it descends through the spinal canal. There are two bulges on the cord, one at the cervical level and the other at the lumbar level, known as the cervical and lumbar nodes. The inner core of the cord in cross-section resembles the letter "H." It is composed of gray matter and comprises what are known as the anterior, posterior, and lateral horns (the terminal ends of the "H"—see Figure 3.3). The white matter portion of the cord, which surrounds the inner core, is composed of band-like structures termed anterior, posterior, and lateral columns. These columns (bundles of nerve fibers arranged vertically in a pillar-like fashion) make up the numerous projection tracts (the connecting nerve fibers) also known as the sensory and motor conduction pathways between the peripheral nervous system and the brain. The pathways are known as the spinal nerves.

The Spinal Nerves

Made up of sensory dendrites and motor axons, and containing the autonomic postganglionic fibers, spinal nerves are classified as mixed nerves. There are thirty-one pairs of spinal nerves, and each nerve in the pair originates from either the anterior or the posterior roots of the spinal cord and emerges through the intervertebral foramina (see Figure 3.4). As they emerge, they branch out and terminate in various parts of the body—the skin, the musculoskeletal structures, and so on. The spinal nerves are not assigned special names, but are merely numbered according to the level of the spinal column from which they emerge (see Figures 8.1 and 8.2 for their distribution). The pairs consist of eight cervical, twelve thoracic, five lumbar, five sacral, and one pair of coccygeal

The Spinal Cord and Central Nervous System Functions 23

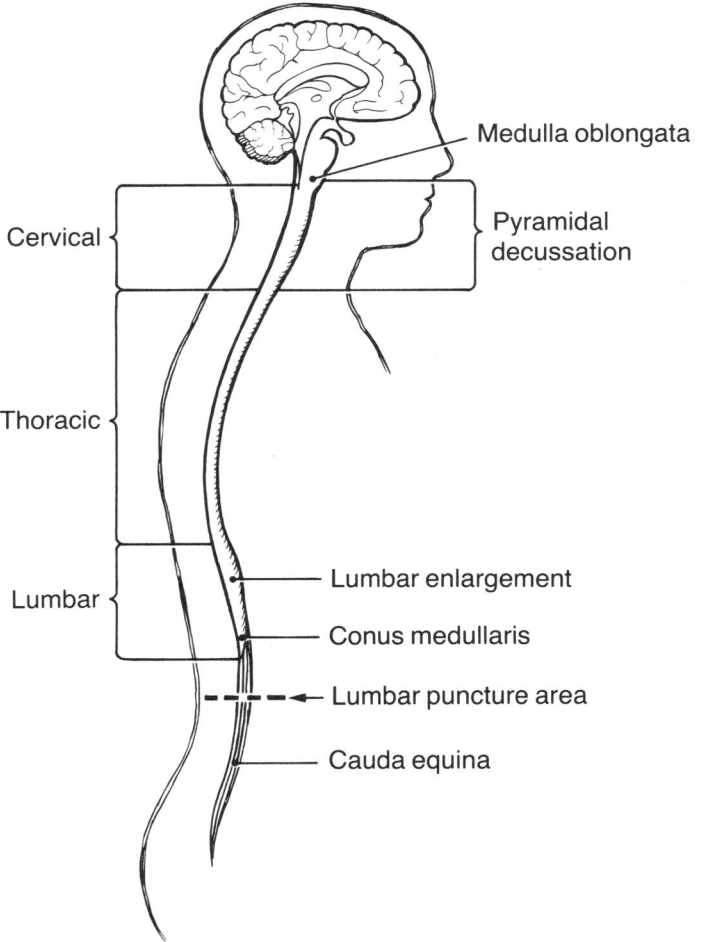

Figure 3.2. Spinal cord levels.

nerves. Through these nerves, which connect the brain to every part of the peripheral nervous system, communication and integration of the human body are achieved.

The human nervous system behaves much like an electrical circuit. As long as there are no interruptions or breaks in the circuit, it will funtion well. However, if an interruption such as frayed wires in the circuit or demyelination of the nerves occurs, their ability to conduct smoothly will be partially or totally dis-

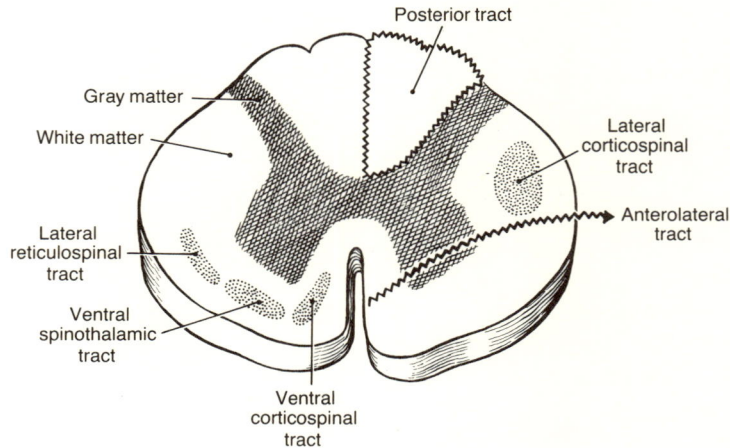

Figure 3.3. Cross-section of spinal cord, showing some of the major spinothalamic tracts.

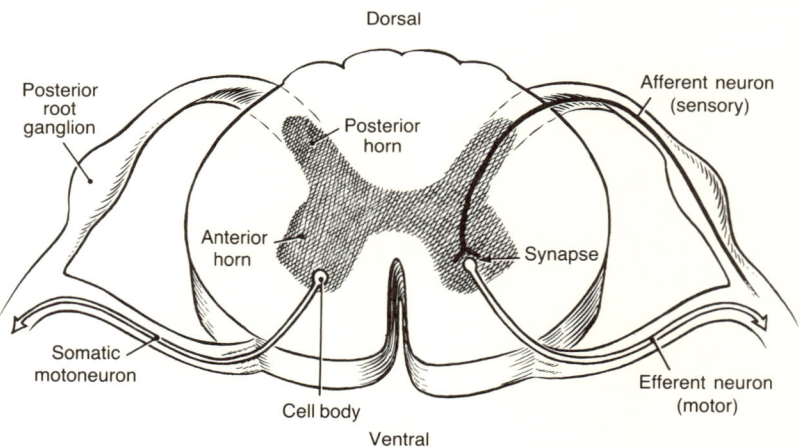

Figure 3.4. Cross-section of spinal cord, including spinal nerves as they exit the cord.

rupted. An electrical circuit disruption will be expressed by a light going on and off intermittently. In the case of the human nervous system, the disruption will be expressed by various degrees of uncontrolled muscular activity or behavioral changes. The behavioral changes may range from a momentary blank stare to sustained bizarre behavioral patterns such as total lack of orientation, compulsive acts, and so on. The muscular abnormality may range from a fine tremor of a small muscle group to generalized grand mal convulsive activity (major motor seizure), depending on the location and severity of the interruption in impulse conduction (definition of various types of seizures can be found in the glossary at the end of the book).

Spinal Tap

The spinal tap is performed between the third and fourth lumbar vertebral spaces for diagnostic and therapeutic purposes. It is done under strict aseptic conditions. A sterile field for the equipment is created by a three- to five-minute surgical scrub of the area followed by an antiseptic spray application. The diagnostic purposes for a tap are:

1. to measure the cerebrospinal fluid (CFS) pressure,
2. to obtain CSF for visualization and laboratory examination,
3. to perform spinal fluid dynamics for signs of blockage caused by tumors or other pathological conditions of the spinal cord, and
4. to inject air, oxygen, or radiopaque substances for radiographic visualization of the nervous system (that is, a myelogram).

The therapeutic purposes of a spinal tap are:

1. to remove blood or pus from the subarachnoid space,
2. to inject drugs and sera,
3. to reduce intracranial pressure, and
4. to administer spinal anesthesia.

There are several contraindications—situations when a spinal tap should not be performed or should be aborted after its start. They are:

1. If the tap does not aid in diagnosis or treatment of the illness.
2. When an intracranial tumor or hemorrhage is suspected and there is clinical evidence of greatly increased intracranial pressure. (Clinical signs may include sudden or unexplained rise in systemic blood pressure, severe headache, bounding pulse, vertigo, loss of balance, dilation of one or both pupils, loss of consciousness with blowing respirations, facial drooping, and papilledema.)
3. When there is evidence of an infection at the tap site.
4. If there is a myelogram or spinal anesthesia administration contemplated within a day or two.

The last two contraindications are to avoid repeated punctures within a short space of time. The tap should be aborted if the CSF pressure is greater than 180 mm H_2O even after relaxing the patient's legs, or if the CSF remains bloody after the first few cc's (the first few cc's may be bloody due to a traumatic tap), or the patient's clinical condition deteriorates suddenly.

The normal opening pressure of CSF should be 60 to 180 mm H_2O. If it is less than 60 mm, it is indicative of blockage above the tap site, which may be in the spinal cord or ventricles in the brain. If the pressure is greater than 180 mm, it is indicative of increased intracranial pressure (ICP).

To prepare for a spinal tap:

1. Place the patient in a lateral recumbent position. The back should be as near to the edge of the bed as possible, with the legs flexed on the thighs, and the thighs on the abdomen and the shoulders and head bent toward the knees. This bowing of the spine will afford the greatest space between the vertebrae.
2. Prep the skin with Betadine or Phisohex (scrub an eight-inch area for three to five minutes) and spray with Merthiolate.
3. Assist the physician as necessary. Help the patient maintain the correct position and observe his tolerance of the procedure. Take vital signs, pre- and post-tap.
4. Make the patient comfortable after the tap is completed, dispose of the equipment, submit the samples to the laboratory, and complete the patient's chart. The charting should

The Spinal Cord and Central Nervous System Functions

include the date, time, physician's name, the level of the tap, opening and closing pressures, gross appearance of the samples, the patient's tolerance and vital signs, and the tests ordered (and the nurse's signature).

Common tests on CSF and the normal values are:

Appearance	Clear and colorless
Red blood cells	None
White blood cells	0–5 cells/mm^3 (agranulocytes)
Protein	15–45 mg / 100 ml
Glucose	40–80/100 ml (60–80 percent of current blood glucose level)
Microorganisms	None

Common conditions which may alter the above values are:

A *bloody sample* is indicative of cerebral hemorrhage or trauma.

A *xanthrochromic* (yellowish) *sample* is indicative of an excessive amount of broken down red blood cells or bilirubinemia and may be due to subarachnoid hemorrhage occurring 3 to 28 days previously.

A *turbid* (milky or cloudy) *sample* may be indicative of high white cell count or high protein or sugar. These may result from a viral or bacterial infection such as meningitis or from encephalitis, space-occupying lesions, brain abcess, multiple sclerosis, mastoiditis, and a number of other conditions.

The *colloidal gold curve,* which is a qualitative and quantitative study of the protein levels within the spinal fluid, helps to determine the presence of specific diseases such as tubercular meningitis, poliomyelitis, and encephalitis lethargia. In most cases tabes dorsalis can be identified and, in rare cases, diagnosis of multiple sclerosis can be substantiated.

SENSORY NEURAL PATHWAYS

A sensory neural pathway to the cerebral cortex consists of a chain of at least three sensory neurons designated as I, II, and III. The sensory neuron I of the relay conducts from the periphery to the spinal cord, where it synapses with sensory neuron II. Sensory neuron II then conducts the impulse from the cord (or the brainstem, if we are considering the cranial nerves) up to the thalamus, where it synapses with sensory neuron III. Sensory neuron III then conducts the impulse from the thalamus to the general sensory area of the cerebral cortex. Crude awareness of the sensation occurs when the sensory impulse (conducted by sensory neuron II) reaches the thalamus. The person is aware of a sensation—heat, cold, and so on—but full consciousness of the sensation occurs only when it reaches the cerebral cortex via sensory neuron III. When it reaches the cerebral cortex, the individual can not only identify the sensation correctly, but can discriminate the intensity of it as well. For the most part, the sensory pathways to the cerebral cortex are crossed or decussate pathways. Stimuli originating from the right side of the body will reach the left side of the cerebral cortex and vice versa. This crossover takes place somewhere in the sensation's ascent to the thalamus via the axon of sensory neuron II. Most sensory neurons form synapses with many other neurons located at various levels of the spinal cord and brain. This interconnection, which is known as the divergence principle, has the important function of making it possible for the nerve impulse to be initiated on more than one receptor and to be conducted to many different effector sites simultaneously, or almost simultaneously.

The function of the neural pathways is to conduct all the varying kinds of impulses between the peripheral nervous system and the brain. The *lateral spinothalamic* pathway, for example, conducts the sensation of pain and temperature, while the *medial lemniscal* and the *ventral spinothalamic* pathways conduct the sensation of touch and pressure.

It is necessary to say a few words about the medial lemniscus system. It is composed of the tracts that make up the posterior white column of the spinal cord, and it includes the *fasciculi cuneatus* and *gracilis*. It is made up of a flat band of white fibers extending through the medulla, pons, and midbrain. These white fibers are composed of axons of sensory neurons II, as in the case of the spinothalamic tracts.

The function of the medial lemniscus system is to transmit impulses that produce our refined discriminatory ability to interpret touch and pressure. This is better known as *stereognosis*—the ability to distinguish the size, shape, and texture of an object.

Another function is localization awareness—the sense of the exact location of a stimulus. In addition, this system provides us with our kinesthetic orientation—our perception of our body's relation to space.

MOTOR NEURAL PATHWAYS

Much is known—and much is still unknown—about the motor neural pathways leading to the skeletal muscles. The discussion of the complex system will be limited to two of its major characteristics. The first is the final *common path*. A motor neural pathway is composed of the motoneurons whose dendrites and cells lie in the anterior gray horn of the spinal cord, and all impulses must traverse through this final path to the skeletal muscles. Therefore, any condition that damages the anterior horn neurons enough to block the conduction of impulses will result in paralysis of the associated muscle. A familiar example is poliomyelitis, a disease that can destroy anterior horn neurons.

Convergence is the second characteristic. This simply means that axons of many neurons converge or synapse with each lower motoneuron so that the impulses from many diverse sources come together, and their combined or summation effect controls the motor pathway functions.

Motor pathways from the cerebral cortex down to the anterior horn motoneurons are many and complex, and there are two methods employed in classifying them. One is based on the location of the fibers in the medulla, and the other on their influence on the lower motoneurons. The first method divides them into pyramidal and extrapyramidal tracts, and the second classifies them as to facilitatory or inhibitory tracts.

Pyramidal tracts are those whose fibers come together in the medulla to form the pyramids—hence their name. Because axons composing the pyramidal tracts originate from neuron cell bodies located in the cerebral cortex (believed to be primarily of *Betz-cells*, large pyramidal ganglion cells forming one of the layers of the motor area of the gray matter of the brain), pyramidal tracts are also called corticospinal tracts. These fibers terminate at various levels of the cord in synapses with interneurons which, in turn, synapse with anterior horn neurons. More than two-thirds of these fibers decussate in the lateral corticospinal tract on the opposite side. The remaining one-third of the fibers, called direct pyramidal tracts, do not decussate but extend down in the ventral corticospinal tract on the same side of the cord as their origin in the cerebral motor area. Impulses over these tracts stimulate the anterior horn cells, which, in turn, stimulate individual muscles, namely of the hands and feet, to produce small discrete movements. The example, mentioned before, of tying one's shoelaces is an act controlled by direct pyramidal tract stimulation. If there is an interruption at any point in the pyramidal tracts, these movements cannot be performed and paralysis may be evident. This is the case following a cerebral vascular accident (CVA), where paralysis occurs due to injury to or pressure on (a) the pyramidal tract's neurons, (b) their cell bodies in the motor area, or (c) their axons of the internal capsules. The internal capsule is located between the thalamus and the caudate and lentiform nuclei in the interior of the cerebrum and is composed of white matter containing a group of sensory and motor projection tracts.

Extrapyramidal tracts are much more complex than the pyramidal tracts. They make up all the pathways between the motor cortex and anterior horn cells with the exception of the pyramidal tracts. The upper extrapyramidal tracts relay impulses between the cerebral cortex, basal ganglia, thalamus, and brainstem.

The lower extrapyramidal tracts conduct impulses that facilitate large, automatic movements and also control automatic facial expressions and movement accompanying many emotions, such as the smile or frown. A smile happens automatically if something pleases us, a frown when something affects us adversely.

The lower extrapyramidal tract (or reticulospinal tract) originates from cell bodies in the reticular formation of the brainstem and terminates in the gray matter of the spinal cord, where it synapses with interneurons, which, in turn, synapse with lower motoneurons. Some of these reticulospinal fibers contain facilitatory tracts, while others make up the inhibitory tracts.

The facilitatory tracts have a stimulating effect on the anterior horn cells by decreasing the neurons' resting potential and initiating impulse conduction. They tend to increase the tone of the extensor muscles and decrease the tone of the flexor muscles, as well as helping to maintain normal muscle tone. The facilitatory impulses under normal conditions slightly exceed the inhibitory impulses. In diseased states, however, this condition is reversed and rigidity or spasticity develops. Parkinson's disease and strokes (CVAs), for example, may interrupt transmission of these impulses. "Pyramidal signs"—notably a spastic type of paralysis, exaggerated deep reflexes, and a positive Babinski's reflex—are the result of interruption in impulse conduction in both the pyramidal and the extrapyramidal inhibitory pathways. Paralysis is more indicative of interruption to the pyramidal tract, whereas spasticity (rigidity) and exaggerated deep reflexes are related to the extrapyramidal pathways. On the other hand, flaccid paralysis is the chief sign of impulse blockage (or injury) to the lower motor neurons in the final common pathway.

THE RETICULAR ACTIVATING SYSTEM

An important function of the central nervous system is the arousal or alerting mechanism. There are two theories regarding the state of wakefulness. At one time it was believed that "conscious, wakeful, and alert states could be maintained, if there were sufficient number of sensory impulses that reached the cerebral cortex via the sensory pathways."[*] The generally accepted theory at the present time states that consciousness, or wakeful and alert state, is achieved by impulses reaching the cerebral cortex via the *reticular activating system,* and not the impulses over the sensory pathways.

The reticular activating system (RAS) consists of nuclei in the brainstem in reticular formation and tracts to and from it. Impulses are continually fed into the brainstem's reticular formation by direct spinoreticular tracts and its collaterals from spinothalamic, auditory, and visual sensory tracts. The impulses travel from the reticular formation to the cerebral cortex. The pathways from the brainstem's reticular formation to the cortex are believed to be composed of long, multisynaptic tracts that have relay

---

[*]Catherine Anthony-Parker, *Textbook of Anatomy and Physiology,* 9th ed. (St. Louis: C. V. Mosby, 1975).

stations or tracts to the hypothalamus, thalamus, and other parts of the brain before the final relay reaches the cerebral cortex. If there is an interruption in the reticular activating system, such as blockage, unconsciousness results. General anesthesia is believed to inhibit the reticular activating system's conducting ability, thus causing unconsciousness. On the other hand, drugs such as amphetamines and adrenalin affect the system conversely or produce wakefulness by stimulating the RAS. In addition to the arousal function, RAS serves some motor functions as well.

REFLEXES

A reflex is an action that results from a nerve impulse passing over a reflex arc, or a response to a stimulus, and it is usually an unconscious, uncontrolled activity that does not involve cerebral cortex activity. Here are some of the major reflexes, how to test for them, and their clinical implications in disease states.

Knee Jerk or Patellar Reflex

This reflex produces a stretching or straightening of the lower leg after the tap (stimulus) is applied. It is a two-neuron reflex arc, or monosynaptic arc, since the impulse crosses only one synapse. The reflex arc that activates a knee jerk is located in the spinal cord's gray matter. It is ipsilateral—the impulse that produces the action does not cross over from one side of the body to the other.

Ankle Jerk

The ankle jerk is elicited by tapping the Achilles tendon. It is also an extensor reflex and is mediated by a two-neuron arc located between the first and second sacral segments of the cord (extension of the cord covering).

Babinski Reflex

This reflex, which is an extension of the great toe with or without fanning of the other toes when the outer margin of the sole of the foot is stroked, is abnormal after the age of one and a half years when the corticospinal fibers become fully myelinated. An abnormal or positive Babinski, dorsiflexion of the great toe, is indicative of pyramidal tract lesion.

Corneal Reflex

A winking (blinking) response when the cornea is touched (usually with a wisp of cotton), this reflex is mediated by the sensory fibers in the ophthalmic branch of the fifth cranial nerve, centers in the pons, and motor fibers in the seventh cranial nerve. Absence of the corneal reflex may indicate a pontine lesion or cerebral edema.

Abdominal Reflex

A drawing in of the abdominal wall when the side of the stomach is stroked, this reflex is mediated by arcs within the sensory and motor fibers in the ninth to twelfth thoracic spinal nerves. If the reflex is diminished or absent, a lesion involving the pyramidal tract's upper motor neurons may be present.

Gag and Cough Reflex

Stimulation of the posterior nasopharynx with foreign matter should result in gagging or coughing. This reflex is mediated by the medulla, and the impulse is transmitted by the vagus (tenth cranial) nerve. The danger of aspiration must be considered if these reflexes are not intact (see the following section).

Swallowing or Palatal Reflex

Stimulating the soft palate should result in swallowing. It is also mediated by the medulla, and the impulse is transmitted by the glossopharyngeal (ninth cranial) nerve. Interruption in the conduction pathway of this nerve or disturbance within the medulla interferes with the patient's ability to swallow. The possibility of aspiration must be guarded against by withholding oral food and fluids, positioning the patient on his side, and keeping suctioning equipment at his bedside.

AUTONOMIC NERVOUS SYSTEM

The autonomic nervous system is the part of the system that sends efferent fibers to visceral effectors. Visceral effectors are defined both in terms of tissues and of organs. In terms of tissues, visceral effectors consist of cardiac muscle, smooth muscles, and glandular epithelium. The organs that are known as visceral effectors consist of the heart, blood vessels, iris, ciliary muscles, hair muscles, various thoracic and abdominal organs, and the body's many glands. All these structures are controlled by the autonomic nervous system and are all involuntary or automatic in their functions, which lie outside conscious control. The system is composed predominantly of motoneurons, although sensory neurons also play a part in the autonomic system's functioning. The system operates on the reflex arc principle. A sensory neuron can function in both autonomic and somatic reflex arcs, whereas a motoneuron can function in either arc but not both. The autonomic nervous system has two divisions: the sympathetic, or thoracolumbar, and the parasympathetic, or craniosacral division.

The *sympathetic* division consists of two chains of ganglia located on either side of the spine and fibers that connect with each other and with the thoracic and lumbar segments of the cord. There are also fibers extending out to the viscera. The *parasympathetic* division consists of ganglia located on or near viscera with fibers between ganglia and brainstem, fibers between ganglia and the sacral region of the cord, and fibers extending into the viscera and glands.

The autonomic nervous system contains pre- and post-ganglionic neurons with synapses between them. The pre-ganglionic neurons conduct impulses either from the cord or brainstem—that is, the frontal cortex and the hypothalamus—to autonomic ganglia. Here they synapse with dendrites and cell bodies of the post-ganglionic neurons, which then conduct the impulses from the autonomic ganglia to the visceral effectors. The most fundamental difference between the autonomic neurons and somatic effector innervation is that the autonomic neurons conduct impulses in a relay fashion to the visceral effectors, while the somatic effector pathways conduct impulses via one motoneuron from the central

The Spinal Cord and Central Nervous System Functions   35

nervous system to the skeletal muscles. The sympathetic nervous system also has many collaterals which account for the widespread response (effect) of many organs at once.

The cell bodies of the parasympathetic system's pre-ganglionic neurons reside in nuclei in the brainstem or in the lateral gray columns of the sacral cord. Their axons are contained in the cranial nerves III, VII, IX, X, and XI, and in some of the pelvic nerves.

Dual autonomic innervation applies to the visceral effectors that receive both sympathetic and parasympathetic fibers, including the cardiac muscle, iris, bronchial tubes, the digestive tract, and so on. *Single autonomic innervation* applies to the visceral effectors receiving only sympathetic fibers—for example, the adrenal medulla, sweat glands, most blood vessels, and the muscles of the hairs.

Terminals of autonomic axons, like those of all axons, release chemicals—in this case autonomic chemical transmitters—that transmit impulses across the synapses and neuroeffector (neuromuscular) junctions. The autonomic axons fall into two classes based on the chemical transmitters they release. Some release acetylcholine and are classified as cholinergic fibers. The others release epinephrine and norepinephrine and are classified as adrenergic fibers.

The axons that comprise the cholinergic autonomic fibers are all pre-ganglionic axons, almost all parasympathetic post-ganglionic axons, and a few sympathetic post-ganglionic axons (controlling certain blood vessels and sweat glands). The adrenergic nerve fibers are all sympathetic post-ganglionic axons, although blood vessels and sweat glands, as previously mentioned, have cholinergic fibers.

THE BALANCING FUNCTION OF THE AUTONOMIC NERVOUS SYSTEM

Both sympathetic and parasympathetic impulses continually play on each other, and whichever is the stronger at a given time will predominate. The heart rate, for example, will slow if the parasympathetic system releases more acetylcholine than the sympathetic releases norepinephrine, which tends to accelerate the heart rate. A relatively stable balance is maintained, however, in good health and a calm environment. Under stress the sympathetic nervous system will prevail, with its "fight or flight" response. The instinctual response to stress, if it is perceived as a threat to survival, safety, or happiness, is to attack the stressor or take flight and leave the scene. In the case of jumping out of the way of an oncoming automobile, it is socially acceptable behavior. Hitting one's employee if one is dissatisfied with a worker's productivity level is, of course, not. The stress level may be the same in both cases, however, and the body's response by the release of adrenalin generating extra energy will be the same also. This energy must find expression; if not, stress remains unresolved and psychosomatic disorders will develop. Each individual interprets stress and responds to it differently. Through learned behavior and social adaptation one learns what is acceptable in one's society and conforms to the social norms. If an individual cannot conform to the social norms, he will do one of two things. He will either behave in an unacceptable manner, or he will suppress his anger by internalizing it or turning it against himself. Psychosomatic disorders are generally believed to be a direct result of the internalization of stressful situations, which are expressed in peptic ulcer disease, ulcerative colitis, dependency on alcohol and drugs, and so on. Most, but not all, of the visceral effectors are controlled by the sympathetic nervous system during stress. In the case of peptic ulcer disease, the parasympathetic nervous system is responsible.

Although, as implied by its name, the autonomic nervous system governs autonomous functions—those independent of conscious will—it is not a separate entity or independent of the nervous system in any sense. It is part of it and functions as such with the brainstem as its main control.

We have examined the structures and primary functions of the brain and the spinal cord, and the systems associated with them. The last component of the nervous system—the cranial nerves—will be considered in the next chapter.

CHAPTER 4 | # THE CRANIAL NERVES

Twelve pairs of nerves arise from the undersurface of the brain, some from each division with the exception of the cerebellum. They pass through small foramina in the skull to their respective destinations. They appear in numerical order from front to back and derive their names from their location or their function. These nerves are composed of efferent fibers that originate outside of the brainstem, afferent fibers that originate in the nuclei of the brainstem, and mixed fibers with cell bodies located both within and outside of the brainstem. (An easy aid to recall the cranial nerves by name and sequence as they arise from the brain is the nonsense rhyme "On Old Olympus Tiny Tops/a Finn and German Viewed Some Hops.")* Table 4.1 identifies the cranial nerves by number, function, and location of cell bodies.

HOW TO TEST THE CRANIAL NERVES

The following is a summary of means of testing the cranial nerves, and of the clinical implications of impairment of their functions.

I. The *olfactory* nerve is the nerve for the sense of smell. Have the patient identify various types of odors—the sour smell of vinegar, and so on. The impairment of this nerve does not require special nursing considerations to meet the patient's normal activities of daily living (ADL).

II. The *optic* nerve is the nerve governing vision. The sensory receptor is the retina, from which the nerve fibers run together as the optic nerve. The retina together with the optic nerve head are

*Catherine Anthony-Parker, *Textbook of Anatomy and Physiology*, 9th ed. St. Louis:, C. V. Mosby, 1975.

Table 4.1: The Cranial Nerves

Number	Name	Function	Location
I.	Olfactory	Smell	Nasal mucosa and cortex
II.	Optic	Vision	Retina and thalamus
III.	Oculomotor	Eye movement, regulation of pupil size, and accommodation	Midbrain
IV.	Trochlear	Eye movements	Midbrain
V.	Trigeminal	Face movements and chewing	Pons
VI.	Abducens	Abduction of eye	Pons
VII.	Facial	Taste buds, secretion of saliva, facial expressions	Pons-medulla
VIII.	Acoustic:		
	Vestibular branch	Equilibrium or balance	Pons-medulla
	Cochlear (auditory)	Hearing	
IX.	Glossopharyngeal	Taste, swallowing, saliva production, reflex control of blood pressure and respiration	Medulla
X.	Vagus	Heart rate, peristalsis, muscles for voice production	Medulla
XI.	Spina accessory	Shoulder and head movements, movements of viscera, voice production	Medulla
XII.	Hypoglossal	Tongue movements	Medulla

commonly referred to as the *fundus*. The nerve itself is an extention of the cranial meninges, and an increase in intracranial pressure will press on the nerve head causing it to swell (papilledema). With the aid of an ophthalmoscope, the fundus (optic disc) can be visualized. Without papilledema, the fundus will visualize as a distinct round disc with well-defined arteries and veins. With papilledema the optic disc is indistinct, the blood vessels are engorged, and retinal hemorrhages are common (a condition referred to as chocked optic disc.) The location and severity of the pressure determine how much involvement there is of the visual field. The effect on the visual field may range from partial loss of peripheral side vision to total blindness in the eye. Have the patient look at your index finger and, without moving his eye or head, tell you how far he can see your finger out to the side. If he has lost his peripheral vision, he must be approached directly face to face, his food tray must be arranged within his field of vision to avoid burns resulting from spilled hot liquids, and he will need assistance with ambulation to keep him from bumping into things.

III. The *oculomotor* nerve controls the eyeball's up, down, and inward motion. It also raises the upper eyelid and constricts the pupil in response to direct light. If there is an interruption of the autonomic portion of the *oculomotor* nerve cells, the pupil will not react to light (constrict), although it can converge (focus on an object) and accommodate for near and far vision. This condition is known as the Argyll Robertson pupil. Consensual reflex (response) is another pupillary function said to be present when one eye is shielded from the light during an examination and yet responds to the light as if it were receiving the stimulus. This is a purely reflex action. Examination of pupillary reaction is done in as dark an environment as possible. Close the patient's eyes and open one at a time as you shine the light on the pupil, approaching the eye from the side with the light, then repeat the same with the other eye. The pupils should appear in midline, be equal in size, and range from 3 mm to 4 mm in diameter. Using the Glasgow Coma Scale (GCS), record the findings as to pupillary size, equality, and reaction to light. A notation should also be made as to their briskness or sluggishness, as they may start out normally and change as intracranial pressure increases. A positive sign denotes reaction to light and a negative sign denotes no reaction. Any clinical condition that can cause increased intracranial pressure or paralysis of the eye muscles will alter the pupils in their position, size and/or ability to react to light. Some of these underlying conditions may be due to tissue destruction, expanding volumes from malignancy, or bleeding. Intracranial or intracerebral bleeding such as a CVA will cause the pupil to become dilated and fixed on the opposite side from where the bleeding occurred in the brain tissue. On the other hand, constriction of the pupil results from paralysis of the fiber optic nerves or may be the result of drugs such as morphine. Drugs with anticholinergic properties such as atropine will dilate the pupils.

If the patient is unable to close his eyes or his corneal reflexes (blinking ability) are absent, drying out of the eyeballs and corneal ulceration must be guarded against. This is accomplished by applying eyedrops or eye ointment for lubrication every two hours. If neither is available, eye pads or small dressings soaked in sterile saline solution placed over the eyes with the eyelids taped will serve the same purpose.

IV. The *trochlear* nerve supplies the superior oblique muscles of the eyeball that rotate the eye down and inward.

V. The *trigeminal* nerve is composed of three branches, as its name suggests, and it contains both sensory and motor fibers. Interruption in the motor fibers interferes with the patient's ability to open his mouth or make chewing motions, and his lower jaw will deviate toward the paralyzed side. His nutritional management becomes a nursing challenge. The sensory portion of the trigeminal nerve sends out three branches—the ophthalamic, maxillary, and the mandibular. The *ophthalamic* branch innervates the forehead and its skin, upper eyelids, the cornea, conjunctiva, and part of the nose and its mucous membrane lining. The second or *maxillary* branch innervates the skin of the cheek, the rest of the nose, lower eyelid, upper lip, the buccal mucosa, and the upper teeth. The third or *mandibular* branch innervates the skin of the lower lip, chin, ear, the lower teeth, and the tongue.

To test the trigeminal's first branch, ask the patient to open and close his eyes and wrinkle his nose or forehead. If he is unable to do so, test the corneal reflex by sliding a wisp of cotton across his open eye. Test the second branch by having him smile, purse his lips, or wrinkle his nose, and the third branch by asking the patient to extend his tongue. It should be midline and without tremors. At the time of testing, observation for facial symmetry is also made. If there is any impairment of the second or third branch, the patient's oral intake must be modified. Depending on the severity of the impairment, the patient should be on a soft or liquid diet, or food should be withheld. Functional oropharyngeal suctioning equipment must be available for immediate use.

VI. The *abducens* nerve is purely motor in nature and innervates the lateral rectus muscle of the eyeball, which rotates it outward.

VII. The *facial* nerve is mostly motor, although it has some sensory and autonomic fibers. It innervates the face, part of the ear and nose, the neck, the anterior two-thirds of the tongue and taste buds, the lacrimal, salivary, and parotid glands.

To test the facial nerve, ask the patient to grimace and to identify the taste of salt and sugar with his eyes closed. Then check his tongue and buccal mucosa for dryness. If he is unable to produce tears, eye care must be instituted, as discussed earlier. If he is unable to produce saliva, oral care is mandatory every two hours. Oral care is done by brushing the teeth, followed by the use of mouth wash and a light coat of water-soluble lubricant such as glycerin applied inside the mouth and on the tongue and lips. If the patient is edentulous (without teeth), use a cotton swab dipped in a solution made up of equal parts of mouth wash (Cepecol is one of the best choices), hydrogen peroxide, and normal saline. Be sure that the entire oral cavity and tongue are cleansed before applying the lubricant. Mixing a small amount of lemon juice with glycerin makes it more tolerable to the patient's palate and more refreshing as well. Oral care is given to prevent herpes sordes and inflammation of the parotid glands, which may result in abcess formation and necessitate surgical intervention.

VIII. The *acoustic* nerve is sensory in nature and has two branches, the vestibular and the cochlear branch. The vestibular branch originates in the medulla, but some fibers extend into the cerebellum and terminate in the semicircular canals of the ear. These fibers provide the sensation of balance and kinetic orientation. Loss of balance or equilibrium occurs if there is disruption or increased pressure anywhere along the nerve fiber pathway between the semicircular canal and the cerebellum. Besides loss of balance, muscular coordination, and spatial orientation, the patient may experience severe vertigo and nausea. The patient with equilibrium and balance disturbances must avoid sudden positional changes and will need assistance with ambulation.

To test the *vestibular branch,* the examiner starts with the ear, using an otoscope to visualize the tympanic membrane to exclude the possibility of *otitis media* (inflammation of the middle ear), a condition which can create pressure on the semicircular canals. If the patient is ambulatory, have him tandem-walk, heel to toe, without looking at the floor. Next have him extend his arms out to the sides and with his eyes closed touch the tip of his nose with the right index finger, repeating with the left. Note the degree of difficulty he has with tandem-walking or by how much he misses the tip of his nose. The examiner must be near enough to the patient for assistance should he need it. If the patient is to remain on bed rest, have him flex his right leg at the knee and, starting at the great toe of his left foot, bring his right heel along the edge of his foot and up the left shin, repeating the process on the opposite side. If there is a vestibular problem, he will not be able to trace a path up the shin, and his movement will not be smooth.

The *cochlear branch* of the nerve is concerned with hearing. Again the examination starts with the tympanic membrane—while talking with the patient, notice whether he cups his hand around the external ear for better hearing or tries to lip read. If any hearing impairment is noted, further examination is necessary. Rubbing your index finger and thumb together, have the patient describe the sound and its location while his eyes are closed, for sound identification. For vibratory identification, a tuning fork is used. When it is activated and held midline above the patient's head over the parietal area, ask him where he hears the vibratory sounds. He should hear them equally in both ears. If he does not, further investigation is necessary, and the Rinne test should be performed, as it may be a conduction-related hearing loss. To perform the Rinne test, activate the tuning fork into light vibration, place it with the one prong end on the patient's mastoid process, and hold it there until the patient no longer hears it. Activate the fork again and hold the U-shaped aspect of it near the patient's ear until he no longer hears it. Both these maneuvers must be timed and the time differences noted. Normally the individual will report hearing the sound longer through air than through bone.

In the presence of otitis media, not only may the hearing and balance be affected but the condition may also account for other neurological symptoms, including focal (localized) seizures, facial paralysis on the affected side, intracranial infection, meningitis, or an increased white blood cell count in the cerebrospinal fluid.

IX. The *glossopharyngeal* nerve is composed of motor, sensory, and autonomic fibers. The motor fibers innervate the constrictor muscles of the pharynx, making swallowing possible. The sensory fibers innervate the posterior one-third of the tongue, the soft palate, and the tonsils. The nerve aids in the transmission of taste sensations. The parasympathetic fibers, which terminate in the parotid gland, stimulate saliva production. The autonomic sensory fibers, extending into the carotid sinus, are responsible for lowering blood pressure and pulse rate. Its clinical significance is important in the manual control of paroxysmal atrial tachycardia (PAT): through carotid sinus massage the heart rate can be slowed down and thereby cardiac output improved. A word of caution, however: nurses should never attempt this maneuver, which is done by a physician only. Emergency cardiopulmonary resuscitation equipment must be on hand as the patient may have a cardiac arrest and, of course, the patient's cardiac status is monitored continuously with the readout tape turned on. The tape is saved for record keeping.

X. The *vagus* nerve runs parallel to the glossopharyngeal nerve. Both nerves are composed of mixed nerve fibers, and in part they share the same functions. The vagus motor nerve fibers supply the voluntary control of the pharynx and larynx, and the involuntary control of the esophagus, bronchi, lungs, heart, stomach, small intestines, liver, pancreas, and kidneys. The autonomic sensory nerve fibers of the vagus nerve supply the larynx, trachea, lungs, esophagus, stomach, small intestines, gallbladder, and the aorta as well.

XI. The *spinal accessory* nerve is composed of motor fibers originating in the medulla and in the upper portion of the spinal cord. Those that begin in the medulla terminate in the pharynx and larynx and aid in voice production. The spinal cord fibers innervate the sternocleidomastoid and the upper trapezius muscles, making shoulder and head movement possible. The testing of this nerve involves having the patient shrug his shoulders and turn his head from side to side. *If, however, there is a suspected or confirmed spinal cord injury, this test is not to be attempted.*

XII. The *hypoglossal* nerve fibers are purely motor in nature. They originate in the medulla oblongata and innervate the muscles of the tongue. To test the hypoglossal nerve, ask the patient to extend his tongue; if it is not midline and has a trembling motion, the patient must be protected from possible aspiration or asphyxiation. His diet must be modified, suctioning equipment must be kept at his bedside, and he is to be positioned on his side—never left lying on his back.

A brief mention of eye movement disorders should be made here before moving on to the next topic. Abnormal eye movements include: deviation, divergence, dysconjugate gaze, nystagmus, and the doll's eyes phenomenon.

Deviation of the eyes occurs when the visual axes are out of alignment due to muscular weakness. *Skew* deviation is expressed by a down and inward rotation of the eyeball on the side of the cerebellar lesion, and up and outward deviation of the eyeball on the opposite side from the cerebellar lesion. *Divergence* of the eyes is the inability of the eyes to coordinate their movements fixed on a near point. The examiner starts by holding his index finger about two feet away from the patient's eyes and moves his finger toward the patient's nose, observing whether the eyes are capable of coordinating movement from a distance to a fixed near point. One eye may remain fixed midline and adjust to the near point, while the other eye may roll up or downward from the midline. *Dysconjugate* gaze is the reverse of conjugate eye movements, in which the eyes work in unison or move in the same direction. In the dysconjugate gaze disorder one eye follows the examiner's finger, while the other remains in a fixed stare. *Nystagmus* is an involuntary rapid movement of the eyeball, which may occur in any direction. One or both eyes may be involved. The disorder results from either otitis media, irritation or increased pressure on the third cranial nerve, or cerebellar impairment. To test for the *doll's eyes phenomenon* turn the patient's head from side to side: the eyes will move in the opposite direction from the side the head is turned to. This condition results from disturbances within the mesencephalon (midbrain), which is integrally involved in the regulation of ocular reflexes, eye movements, and righting reflexes (the ability of the eyes to assume optimal position after departure from it has occurred). When examining the eyes, one must note the abnormal movements, the direction of occurrence, the eye involved, and the speed of the movements. All the above conditions may be a direct result of increased intracranial pressure regardless of underlying clinical conditions.

CHAPTER 5 | **INTRACRANIAL PRESSURE**

The normal intracranial pressure (ICP) is 0 to 15 mm Hg or 0.20.4 cm H$_2$O. The conversion of mercurial pressure to water pressure is 1 mm Hg = 1.36 cm H$_2$O. This is an important fact to keep in mind, as the manometer is marked in centimeters and the physician's order may be written in millimeters for the treatment of increased ICP.

Intracranial pressure—the pressure within the skull—is generated by intracranial volume. This volume is comprised of the following: brain tissue, blood, and cerebrospinal fluid (CSF). The direct proportionate relationship existing between the intracranial volume and the intracranial pressure can be expressed by V/P, or volume divided by pressure. If an increase in volume occurs, the pressure will rise, and a decrease in volume will allow the pressure to drop.

Conditions that can increase intracranial volume and thereby the pressure are: edema of the brain tissue (brain water), neoplastic growths, and inflammation. The blood component may expand the volume by hemorrhages, hematomas, hypercarbia (retention of carbon dioxide), and vascular anomalies. The cerebrospinal fluid component may be expanded by hydrocephalus resulting from over-production of fluid, blockage of circulation, or the system's inability to absorb the fluid. All these conditions will increase the volume and the pressure, as there is no room for additional contents within the nondistensible cranial vault. If an increase in volume is to be tolerated without an increase in pressure, some of the intracranial contents must leave the cranial vault. This is accomplished, up to a point, by spatial compensatory mechanisms, which respond to an increase in volume and pressure in three ways:

Intracranial Pressure

1. Cerebrospinal fluid is translocated into the subarachnoid space.
2. Cerebrospinal fluid absorption is increased by the subarachnoid villi.
3. The low pressure venous system is compressed to decrease blood volume.

These mechanisms serve to decrease the intracranial volume, to keep the intracranial pressure (ICP) within normal limits. However, if the increase in volume outstrips the ability of the spatial compensatory mechanisms, the pressure will rise. The amount of rise in pressure determines the type and severity of the neurological symptoms the patient will experience.

When the spatial compensatory mechanisms are exhausted, the ICP suddenly and sharply increases. Increased ICP, in turn, causes further damage to brain tissue in two ways. First it interferes with the blood flow to the brain and the brain's *autoregulation* phenomenon—the process whereby the blood flow to the brain is kept constant, even if the systemic blood pressure changes (within certain limits). Above and below a mean arterial pressure (MAP) of 50 to 150 mm Hg, cerebral perfusion pressure (CPP) will be affected. The following formula describes the relationship between systemic blood pressure and intracranial pressure:

$$CPP = MAP - ICP$$

The cerebral perfusion pressure remains constant when the autoregulatory mechanism is functioning correctly and the mean arterial pressure remains within the autoregulatory limits. *The normal CPP range is 50 to 90 mm Hg.* CPP greater than 90 mm Hg results in the development of cerebral edema, and CPP less than 50 mm Hg results in cerebral ischemia. The most common clinical presentation of cerebral ischemia is simple fainting or syncope.

The second way increased ICP can cause damage to brain tissue is by shifting and distorting the brain tissue by pressing it against the nondistensible cranial vault. This, in turn, results in further decrease of blood flow to the brain and is expressed in focal neurological deficits. When a shift and compression occur in the brainstem affecting the vital centers, as in the case of transtentorial herniation (the downward displacement of the brainstem through the foramen magnum), irreversible neurological damage or death occurs rapidly unless the symptoms are recognized promptly and successfully treated. The signs or symptoms of transtentorial herniation include complaints of neck pain, inability to swallow, and difficulty in breathing. The unconscious patient becomes areflexic, his hyperventilation deteriorates to Cheyne-Stokes respiration, and he will demonstrate decerebrate posturing. Respiratory and cardiac arrest will follow very quickly. The patient's vital signs (blood pressure, pulse, and respiration) must be monitored every five to ten minutes—especially the respiratory rate, rhythm, and depth—if there is an underlying clinical condition that may cause rapidly expanding cerebral volume—such as severe head injury, postoperative craniotomy, and massive or central (within the brainstem) cerebral vascular accident. As the intracranial volume expands the pressure increases, resulting in increased edema. This in turn destroys more brain cells as the blood flow to the brain is decreased. This sets up a cycle expressed in progressive neurological deficit (see Figure 5.1).

The immediate treatment for transtentorial herniation includes sitting the patient in an upright position, avoiding hyperextension of the neck, administering Mannitol 500 cc of the 20 percent solution IV (intravenously) rapidly, and standing by with resuscitative equipment until the physician arrives. Although the morbidity and mortality rate is extremely high even with the best possible treatment and care, early recognition of signs and symptoms through constant observation can aid in the prevention of such tragic outcomes.

In summary, intracranial pressure will be affected by the following:

1. Increased intracranial volume and its distribution
2. Integrity of the cranial vault
3. Cardiac output (25 percent of the total cardiac output goes to the brain)
4. Perfusion (adequate blood flow to all body parts)
5. Autoregulatory mechanism of the brain
6. Hypercarbia—CO_2 retention, which dilates the cerebral vessels, with resulting cerebral edema

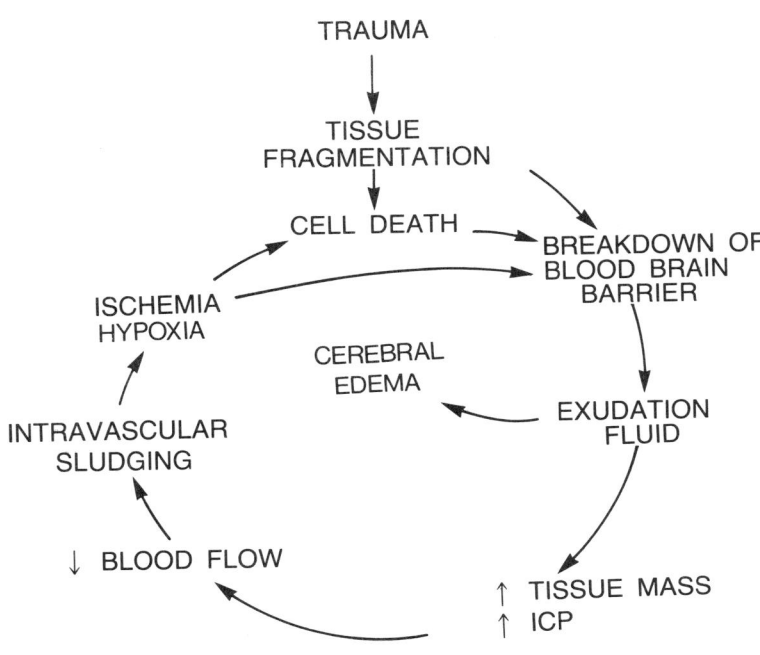

Figure 5.1. Cycle of progressive neurological deficit resulting from evolving cerebral edema.

7. Hypoxia (the brain requires 20 percent more oxygen than any other body organ)
8. REM sleep (rapid eye movements during sleep, believed to be due to stress)
9. Patient's position and activity (rapid head turning or neck flexion may occlude the internal carotids)
10. Emotional and/or painful stimuli
11. Increased intrathoracic pressure—resulting from mechanical ventilation with large tidal volumes. (It is necessary, however, to give 25 ml/kg body weight or 700 to 900 ml per breath to prevent neurogenic pulmonary edema.)

SIGNS AND SYMPTOMS OF INCREASED ICP

1. Headache—localized or diffused
2. Vomiting—usually projectile
3. Vertigo and visual disturbances
4. Papilledema—pupillary changes
5. Mental changes—from slight confusion to deep coma
6. Cardiac changes—slow bounding pulse, elevated blood pressure, and cardiac arrhythmias
7. Respiratory changes—determined by the location and amount of pressure. (Pressure on the pneumotaxic center in the pons will affect the rate and rhythm—ataxic, Biot's, and cluster breathing patterns will result. [See glossary for respiratory patterns.] If the triggering mechanism in the medulla is compressed, hyperventilation, hypoventilation, or apnea will result. Cheyne-Stokes breathing is the result of diffused hemispheric pressure.)
8. Decorticate and decerebrate posturing—late signs (see the following paragraphs).

Decorticate posturing results from increased pressure on the diencephalon. An early sign of pressure is the patient's ability to make slow, aversive movements to painful stimuli. As the pressure increases, however, the patient becomes more immobile and will evidence decorticate posturing. The clinical presentation of decorticate posturing is adduction of the shoulders, flexion at elbows, wrists, and fingers, with hemiplegia and hyperextension (rigidity) of the lower extremities. If the pressure increase is in the lateral hemisphere, contralateral deviation of the eyes away from the hemiplegia is notable (the doll's eyes phenomenon). The tonic deviation of the eye or eyes is not apparent, however, for eight to twelve hours after the occurrence of hemiplegia. If the treatment to reduce increased pressure is not effective, the problem may be an acute pontine lesion. Further neurological deficits, along with respiratory disturbances, will be observable and the patient will become decerebrate.

Decorticate posturing becomes *decerebrate* as the pontine lesion expands, and Cheyne-Stokes respiration changes to neurogenic hyperventilation. Decerebrate posturing may not be evidenced until knuckle pressure is applied to the patient's sternum. To test for decerebrate posturing, place the patient's arms on his abdomen in a semiflexed position and apply knuckle pressure to the midsternum. The patient's response to the sternal stimuli will include internal rotation of the forearm away from the stimuli with fingers flexed and thumbs tucked in between the fingers or into the palms. The pupillary changes are on a continuum from brisk to sluggish to no reaction and dilation.

MONITORING THE INTRACRANIAL PRESSURE

Although physical assessment of the patient's neurological status through observation for subjective clinical signs of increased intracranial pressure is extremely valuable, it cannot give as precise indications as the objective method of observation. Therefore, in addition to subjective observation, intracranial pressure monitoring by mechanical means should be instituted. ICP monitoring is accomplished by insertion of either an epidural probe, a subarachnoid (Richmond) screw, or a retention catheter into the fourth ventricle via a ventriculostomy. The first two devices are useful only in the measurement and reflection of numerical value of the intracranial pressure through the attached transducer. The latter will provide this information and additionally can be used in the treatment to reduce increased pressure by draining off excess CSF. Insertion of these ICP monitoring devices is done by a neurosurgeon via a small twist drill or burr hole. As with any invasive procedure, the possibility of introducing infection exists. The integrity of the drainage system must therefore be preserved and the procedure handled aseptically.

As a rule, in the management of increased intracranial pressure, anything above 20 mm Hg is treated either by draining off CSF via the ventricular catheter or by the use of cerebral dehydrators such as Mannitol, Urea, Lasix, and so on (see the appendix on drugs in common use for dosages and nursing precautions). ICP of up to 100 mm Hg may be left untreated in the patient who has essential intracranial hypertension. With this condition, there is no sudden rise in pressure and associated structural changes as with an acute injury or bleeding episode. As it develops slowly, the patient builds up his tolerance to the high pressure with no neurological impairment, although he may complain of headaches, dizziness, and nausea.

The Glasgow Coma Scale (shown in Figure 5.2) is a useful tool in recording neurological assessment data.

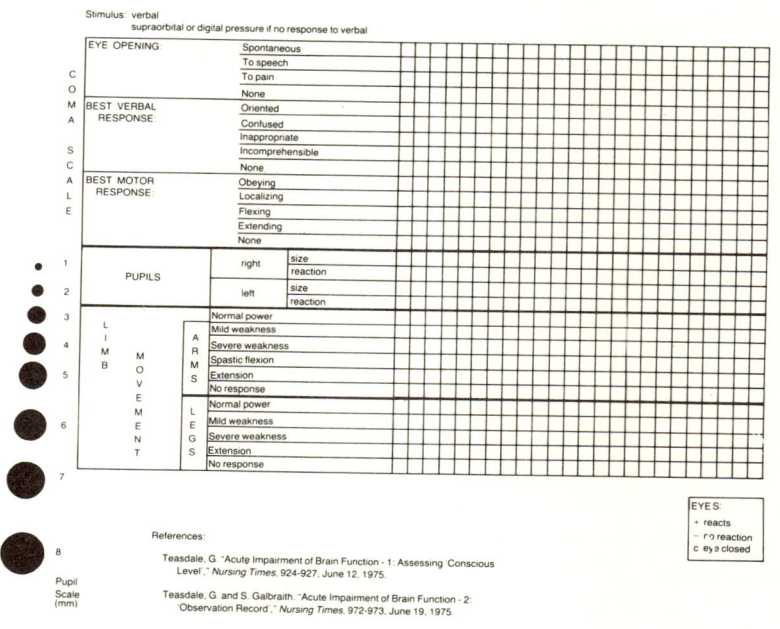

Figure 5.2. Neurological assessment—Glasgow Coma Scale. Adapted from Institute of Neurological Sciences, Glasgow.

CHAPTER 6 | ASSESSMENT OF THE NEUROLOGICAL PATIENT AND THE NURSE'S ROLE IN TREATMENT AND CARE

Neurology is probably one of the most exacting branches of medicine as we know it today. It demands precision and clarity of its practitioners: the physician, the nurse, the radiological technologist, the physical therapist, and any other person with responsibility for the care of the patient with a neurological deficit. It is therefore vital that these health care providers have a sound basic understanding of the anatomy and physiology of the human nervous system and its functions. Furthermore, they must possess keen observational skills, the ability to record gathered data clearly and concisely, knowledge of accepted parameters for the norms, and the ability to recognize any deviations from them, and they must know how to deal with these deviations once they are detected. If the health care providers possess the above qualities and work together as a team, the patient has an improved chance for recovery. If not, he may end up with permanent and needless neurological deficits ranging from a slight paresis or drooping of the face to total paralysis, or he may even die unnecessarily.

NEUROLOGICAL ASSESSMENT

Although the patient may not be entering the hospital with a specific or known neurological deficit, the registered nurse performs a limited neurological examination as part of the admission physical assessment.

In order to collect as much basic information as possible on the patient's condition and general health, a history is taken and a general physical examination is done on each patient at the time of admission to the hospital. Through this routine history and physical, the nurse can learn many things about the patient's neurological status. She can observe the following without any clinical aids: the patient's general health, size, obvious problems, attire, grooming, manner, behavioral patterns, facies, gait, posture, voice, and, above all, his communicative abilities.

In evaluating the patient's communicative abilities, the nurse must consider the three major categories of cerebral cortical functions: *sensory integration, motor integration,* and *language abilities.* Through an assessment of sensory integration, agnosia, apraxia, and aphasia can be detected. The sensory assessment includes functions such as sound identification; auditory-verbal integration; verbalization; written communication; and cognitive capacities such as memory, recall, comprehension, and cooperational abilities. The nurse will evaluate the patient's emotional status by observing body tension, personality traits, affect, mood, appropriateness of response, and comments about the situation at hand. Extremes of emotions may be indicative of neurological disorders. Inappropriate crying and laughing, for example, are common behavioral patterns in patients with pseudobulbar palsy. This type of symptom may also be due to head injury, brain damage, or frontal lobe disease. Evidence of progressive behavioral or cognitive deterioration may indicate the presence of organic cerebral disease. In this latter case, the patient may not even be aware of it, and "little oddities" in behavior may be picked up by the nurse from family members or significant others. If such people are not available, the nurse must ask specific questions to which she knows the correct answers. If, for example, a patient's family states that "he has been misplacing things lately and simply cannot remember what he has done with them," the nurse can easily verify this information by asking the patient to read the last three numbers on his hospital identification band and memorize them, and asking him in ten minutes to repeat these numbers without referring to them again. If he is unable to remember them, he is having short-term memory loss and will be unable to learn new material or follow instructions unless they are repeated each time he is to perform them. This information must be incorporated into the patient's care plan to enable other care providers to meet the patient's needs more efficiently.

Along with behavioral assessment, intellectual capacities and memory are tested. Intellectual capabilities are estimated and are based on vocabulary range, fund of knowledge, life achievements, and educational preparation. Memory is tested while the patient gives his or her history, which covers both recent and more distant memory with questions such as, Have you ever been hospitalized before? When and why? What is your age and birth date? Other questions that may be asked are, What is the name of the hospital you are in? What is today's date? Who is the president of the United States? And so on.

By looking at the patient while gathering historical data, the nurse can observe motor integration, facial expressions, involuntary movements, and the movement and appearance of the eyes. Is the range of vision normal, or does the patient have to turn his head to look at the interviewer? Are there odd or peculiar movements, mannerisms, or tics? Are there any striking physical deformities—wasting or unequal muscle mass size, limpness or drooping? Is there difficulty in maintaining normal posture while walking or sitting? Are there scars, old burns, or multiple bruises? These may be indicative of sensory impairment as well as motor impairment.

The autonomic nervous system can be evaluated by examining the skin for its general appearance with emphasis on color, temperature, and wetness. Questioning the patient on bowel and bladder habits or control, and any problems with the reproductive system, can give important information.

For a complete neurological nursing evaluation, the nurse should have the same equipment that is normally employed for routine physicals, with the addition of a penlight, cotton wisps, cotton-tipped applicators, otoscope, percussion hammer, tuning fork, paper and pencil, sugar and salt, and a sharp (sterile) needle. Such an examination will, of course, provide a very limited neurological assessment—any deficit detected at this juncture can only be put into a broad category of neurological disorders. Further specific, and at times, lengthy testing is needed to identify it definitively for the purpose of diagnosis and treatment. After the initial recognition of an existing problem, the physican should be alerted and the nurse should document the suspected deficit on the patient's records, using precise and descriptive language. The nurse then assists the physician in further testing procedures and is responsible for administering medications as ordered and observing the patient's reactions to both the procedures and medications or treatments. It is extremely critical to record and report even the slightest changes in the patient's clinical condition. This cannot be overemphasized.

INJURIES TO THE CENTRAL NERVOUS SYSTEM

At the present time, more than 100,000 persons in the United States, mostly young people, have sustained spinal cord injuries resulting in para- or quadriplegia. The three major causative factors are vehicular collisions, diving mishaps, and other accidents such as falls from heights. Less serious spinal injuries result from lifting heavy objects, minor falls, or wrenching of the back. This latter category of spinal injuries is seen in the emergency department, but is not admitted to the intensive care unit. The treatment modality is conservative medical management, which may include pelvic traction, bed boards, heat, massage, and muscle relaxers.

Vehicular collisions are responsible for about 70 percent of all head injuries, and again these patients typically are young, about 80 percent of them being between the ages of 15 and 45 years. The majority of these collisions—60 to 80 percent—are due to or directly related to the use of alcohol. The remaining 20 percent of head injuries are caused by acts of violence and falling from heights, with a very small percentage due to contact sports.

Recovery from the injury depends largely on those who care for them, and time is of great importance in initiating the proper care of these patients. Prompt treatment is essential because it is not only the direct injury to the spine and skull that affects recovery. Morbidity and mortality are increased by subsequent edema of the brain and spinal cord, dislocation of the fractured vertebrae of the spine, depressed skull fractures, and collection of blood in the nondistensible cranial vault. *The first twelve to twenty-four hours after the injury have been designated as the most critical period, during which permanent damage to the spinal cord and brain may be prevented, arrested, or reversed.*

EVALUATING THE LEVEL OF CONSCIOUSNESS

The symptoms of patients suspected or known to have sustained a head injury are so variable that unless the patient is unconscious, no specific or typical picture of his clinical state exists. The patient who has no apparent injury but has sustained a blow to the head, which may or may not have been followed by a period of confusion or momentary loss of consciousness, may seem normal upon arrival at the hospital, but may slowly or rapidly deteriorate depending on the severity of the injury. This patient requires the same close observation as the patient who presents in the unconscious state, with the exception that his need for attention is less immediate and his/her treatment may not be as extensive. Treatment and nursing care may range from observation overnight to a craniotomy, followed by long and intensive care in the acute care setting and a period in a rehabilitative facility after the acute phase of the illness has passed.

The cardinal sign of insufficient cerebral function is an alteration of behavior ranging from mild confusion to deep coma, depending on the amount of rise in ICP. Many conditions other than trauma to the head can bring about unconsciousness (coma). The many causes of unconsciousness are divided into three broad categories: (a) those within the central nervous system (CNS), (b) metabolic or toxic factors that affect the nervous system, and (c) exogenous materials that also affect the CNS. The first category includes such conditions as brain tumors, hemorrhage, abcess, stroke, encephalitis, epilepsy, trauma to the brain or adjacent structures, meningitis, and increased intracranial pressure (ICP) regardless of the cause. The second category, metabolic or toxic causes, includes advanced uremia, diabetic acidosis, hypoglycemia, hepatitis, respiratory acidosis, anoxia, hyperventilation, hypertensive encephalopathy, eclampsia, and marked changes in acid-base balance. The most common cause of admission with deep coma in the United States under the third category is intentional or accidental poisoning by ingestion of chemicals such as barbiturates, tranquilizers, insulin, or alcohol. Other exogenous causes are inhalation of carbon monoxide, snake bites, or antigens produced by an anaphylactic reaction. All the above conditions can and will bring about an altered state of alertness, or level of consciousness. The level of consciousness may vary depending on the cause of the condition, time lapse, or the effectiveness of the medical management of the underlying cause.

The following are steps in evaluating stages of altered consciousness. The first step is to evaluate the level of alertness and orientation, which is expressed in three spheres: the recognition of one's self (by name), recognition of place, and orientation to time. If the patient can spontaneously and with reasonable speed respond to questions in these three categories, he is said to be alert and oriented, or oriented X3. If, however, he has trouble with these basic questions, he is said to be obtuse or confused. The next step, as consciousness decreases, is *somnolence,* in which the patient is excessively drowsy and responds by mumbling or making uncoordinated movements when touched. In *stupor,* his response will be to grimace and withdraw from painful stimuli only. In coma, there is no reaction to verbal or painful stimuli and the patient cannot be aroused; he is said to be in a deep coma. In this condition, gag and corneal reflexes are also absent; however, there may or may not be pupillary response to light.

Regardless of the cause of the altered state of consciousness, the end result is an expression of increased intracranial pressure (ICP) due to the expanding volume within the cranium. Increased ICP may be from edema caused by acidotic, anoxic, or toxic states, from bleeding into the brain tissue and overproduction of fluid, or blockage of the cerebrospinal fluid (CSF) circulation. The clinical manifestations will be much the same, with very little variation.

MONITORING AND TREATMENT OF THE UNCONSCIOUS PATIENT

The nursing care of the unconscious patient will include the following:

1. Maintenance of adequate ventilation by whatever means is necessary (brain anoxia longer than five minutes will cause irreversible brain damage and brain death).
2. Establishment of a patent intraveneous line (18 gauge IV device).

3. Monitoring of BP, P, R, and pupillary reaction to light, size, and position Q 15 minutes times 24 hours, then every one hour unless clinical condition or doctor's orders indicate otherwise.
4. Temperature measurement Q 1 to 2 hours (rectal).
5. Accurate hourly intake and output.
6. Careful observation, recording, and immediate reporting of the minutest changes.
7. Interviewing family or others who can contribute to the establishment of the underlying cause.
8. Aiding the physician in diagnostic studies as necessary.

The primary concern for the nurse is to ensure adequate ventilation by whatever means is necessary, as anoxia resulting from inadequate ventilation is the most frequent cause of additional damage to the unconscious patient.

Signs of inadequate ventilation include inadequate respiratory effort with absent or decreased chest or diaphragmatic motion, rate, and depth; cyanosis from inadequate gas exchange (cynosis is a late sign, however); and abnormal arterial blood gases (ABGs). Normal values for ABGs on room air are pH 7.35–7.45, PCO_2 35–45 mm Hg, PO_2 80–98 mm Hg; and HCO_3 22–26 mEq/liter. Certain respiratory patterns are also significant. Cheyne-Stokes respiration is indicative of congestive heart failure or uremia and is frequently a preterminal respiratory effort. Biot's respiration is common in central nervous system disease, especially meningitis.

The next step is to monitor the blood pressure and pulse. Hypertension is commonly seen with conditions that increase intracranial pressure, such as subdural hematoma, strokes, and hypertensive encephalopathy. Hypotension is common in fluid and electrolyte loss accompanying diarrhea, vomiting, burns, or any conditions causing shock. Shock may be caused by circulating volume loss, cardiac pump failure, or loss of vascular resistance due to severe pain, bacteremia, or toxins. Tachycardia may be due to shock, congestive heart failure, high fever, severe hyperthyroidism, and exhaustion. Bradycardia is indicative of increased ICP, Adams-Stokes syncope, simple fainting, and so on. These are a few examples of the many conditions and symptoms that the nurse may encounter in dealing with the unconscious patient.

The pulse is to be taken apically and evaluated for rate, rhythm, and intensity. As the pressure increases on the reticular formation within the medulla oblongata, the pulse will become slow and bounding, as is common in stroke victims.

The temperature is to be taken rectally for accurate core temperature. An elevation may indicate infection, dehydration, or brainstem damage—specifically of the hypothalamus. Hypothermia, on the other hand, may be noted following exposure and overdoses of depressant drugs, such as barbiturates and tranquilizers.

Pupillary dilation, constriction, or unequality indicates the disruption of impulses in the descending fibers from the corticomesencephalic area. These fibers extend to between C1 (the first cervical) to T1 (the first thoracic vertebral) levels from the brainstem via the autonomic nervous system.

Diagnostic studies routinely employed to determine the underlying cause of unconsciousness include complete blood count (CBC), blood sugar, blood urea nitrogen (BUN), serum CO_2, and other electrolytes, and appropriate enzyme studies if the cause is suspected to be cardiac or hepatic in nature. Radiographic studies include chest X-ray to rule out pneumothorax or pleural effusion, skull X-ray to rule out increased ICP or occult head injury, and CAT scan to establish location and size of the brain lesion. A lumbar puncture is frequently done, as has been discussed earlier.

The management of the unconscious patient is symptomatic once the baseline of vital signs has been obtained and cardiac and ventilatory adequacy ensured. By careful observation and alertness to changes in the patient's condition, the nurse makes an important contribution that can assist the physician in establishing the correct diagnosis and choice of treatment.

Systematic observation should include examination of the skin and mucous membranes. Clues to the underlying possible causes of unconsciousness include the following:

1. Multiple needle marks or venipuncture sites, indicative of diabetes or a drug addiction.
2. Poor skin turgor (flabby and dry skin), denoting severe dehydration, electrolyte imbalance and/or acid-base disturbance.

Assessment of the Neurological Patient

3. Extreme diaphoresis, which may be due to severe hypoglycemia (blood sugar less than 30 mg/dl).
4. Pallor and coolness of the skin with a patient in shock, which may indicate internal bleeding.
5. Anasarca, or generalized edema, which may be due to kidney disease or anaphylactic shock.
6. Localized edema, which may be from trauma, even though there is no initial discoloration (especially if the injury was done with a blunt object).
7. Rubor (extremely flushed), which may be indicative of hypertension, alcoholism, or carbon monoxide poisoning.
8. Cyanosis, indicating inadequate oxygenation or poor tissue perfusion.
9. Jaundice, which may accompany coma due to hepatic failure.
10. Hematoma, which is evidence of external injury.
11. Petechiae, which may be seen in the Waterhouse-Friderichsen syndrome in meningococcemia.
12. Uremic frost, which may indicate kidney failure.

Head and neck examination should include pupillary responses, as discussed earlier, with alertness to any changes that may be developing—from brisk to sluggish response, from equal to unequal size. Keep in mind that almost all patients with metabolic coma retain their pupillary reflex to light. The nose and ears should be observed for any drainage and its character—purulent, bloody, serosanguinous, or clear. Clear drainage from the nose or ears may indicate leakage of cerebrospinal fluid, which is seen in basilar skull fractures. Irrigation of the ears is not to be attempted, but a sterile dressing should be placed in the ear and changed as necessary. The odor of the breath may reveal ketoacidosis, intoxication, uremia, or internal bleeding. Resistance to neck movements (nuchal rigidity) is indicative of meningitis or cerebral hemorrhage. *Neck movements are never to be attempted if there is any possibility of cervical spinal injury.*

SUPPORTIVE TREATMENT AND NURSING CARE

The unconscious patient is never to be left unattended and lying on his back. He is to be under the constant supervision of a qualified health care provider and preferably positioned on his side, especially until gastric intubation is instituted. This is to prevent aspiration of vomitus, as projectile vomiting is common with increased intracranial pressure. He is to be maintained in proper body alignment to prevent foot and wrist drop and other contractures. Skin care and turning, using a turn sheet, are mandatory every two hours. All joints should be manipulated through their full range of motion if the period of unconsciousness is prolonged. If unconsciousness persists, a nasogastric tube is inserted first to decompress the stomach and later to provide for more adequate nutritional management. Oral and eye care is the next nursing consideration—it should be attended to every two to four hours. For oral care, use toothpaste and brush, or if the patient is edentulous, use mouthwash with swabs and suction, as discussed earlier. If the patient clenches his jaw, apply pressure to the temporomandibular joint on the side of each cheek to open his mouth. A light application of vaseline is permissible to the lips to avoid dryness, but an excess is to be avoided as it may be inhaled and lead to the development of lipidpneumonia. For eye care, you may use artificial tears, lacrilube, or saline eye pads to prevent corneal ulceration.

Elimination of urine may be facilitated by an indwelling catheter, and the bowels are managed by administration of cathartics or enemas, as ordered.

The nurse should always remember that the patient may hear although he is unable to respond. Therefore, all conversation at the patient's bedside should be as if he were conscious. Remember to talk to your patient while taking care of him, telling him what you are doing and why. It is surprising what he may remember and relate when he recovers.

THE CONVULSING PATIENT

Convulsions can be a manifestation of many different illnesses. As in the management of the unconscious patient, the primary focus is on supporting the vital functions until a definitive diagnosis is made and treatment is instituted. Convulsions, or seizures, may occur in various disordered states including epilepsy, uremia, severe brain trauma, hypoxia, toxemia, tetanus, poisonings, meningitis, encephalitis, diabetic acidosis, marked hypoglycemia, acute alcoholism, alcoholic withdrawal, drug intoxications, increased intracranial pressure, inadequate cerebral perfusion due to low cardiac output, and in any illness capable of causing high fever. The most common cause of a single seizure in children is a febrile state. The convulsing patient who is seen in the emergency department is not always hospitalized and, if hospitalized, may not go to the intensive care unit. The convulsing patient admitted to the intensive care unit is usually having seizures of unknown etiology or presenting *status epilepticus* (repeated seizures that cannot be controlled).

When confronted with a seizing patient, the nurse should keep calm; the seizure cannot be stopped once it is started. The treatment is directed toward the prevention of recurring seizures. Support vital functions as necessary: loosen clothing and roll the patient on his side to facilitate airway maintenance and prevention of aspiration. Do not force anything into his mouth (as the old rule stated.) Do not try to revive him if he stops breathing momentarily; however, supplemental oxygen by mask can be held near the patient's face. The most important thing is to note the onset and/or the duration and the type of muscular activity involved and, of course, to take steps to prevent recurrence. It is normal for the patient to be tired, sleepy, or confused in his post-ictal state. He should be left to rest for at least two hours and may be released from the emergency department after full recovery. If he is a known epileptic, he should be encouraged to see his physician because he may need his medication readjusted. If, however, the patient has no history of seizure disorder and no immediate medical reason is identified for his seizure, he must be admitted.

To manage repeated seizures, phenobarbital, Dilantin, paraldehyde, or Valium should be used, and the patient should be seen by a competent neurologist for a complete workup, especially if status epilepticus develops. If large doses of intravenous Dilantin are administered, the patient must be placed on a cardiac monitor. In rare cases, to control acute convulsive states, the use of Amytal or sodium pentothal is necessary. For febrile seizures, antipyretics are also used.

There are four types of epileptic seizures commonly recognized:

the *petit mal* or minor motor, the *psychomotor,* the *Jacksonian* or focal, and the *grand mal* or major motor. The petit mal (minor motor) seizure's symptom is a transitory loss of consciousness lasting only a second or two and expressed by a vacant or blank stare. It does not incapacitate the individual and often goes unnoticed. A psychomotor seizure is characterized by repetitive activities, performed automatically, which may or may not be appropriate. The individual is not aware of these automatic repetitive activities at the time, nor can he recall them after the seizures. The Jacksonian (focal) seizure is usually a repetitive unilateral involuntary contraction of specific small muscle groups that may spread through one side of the body. It always begins in the same muscle or muscles, such as in the thumb, and follows the same pattern, spreading toward the head first, then toward the leg. The grand mal (major motor) seizure is characterized by repetitive forceful clonic muscle contractions involving the entire body with loss of consciousness, and may include loss of bowel and bladder control. In the post-ictal phase, the patient is confused or amnesiac and is very tired. He will complain of severe muscular aching and may be bleeding from the mouth from having bitten his tongue.

An electroencephalogram (EEG) will be done in addition to the diagnostic laboratory studies normally ordered for the unconscious patient. The EEG may or may not show an abnormal brain wave pattern. The laboratory data and nursing observation, therefore, along with the patient's history, are important for establishment of the underlying cause and choosing the correct modality of medical management.

CHAPTER 7 | HEAD INJURIES

Since the symptoms of patients with head injuries will vary with the severity of the injury and the time lapse between the injury being sustained and time of arrival in the hospital, no typical clinical picture can be presented. The patient may be asymptomatic upon arrival and deteriorate neurologically thereafter, or he may be brought to the hospital in a state of unconsciousness. He may or may not be convulsing or showing signs of decerebration (posturing).

OPEN HEAD INJURIES

Head injuries may be classified as open or closed. A patient with an open injury requires special attention. An open injury, one that penetrates the skull, produces obvious injury to the brain or its supporting structures, such as the meninges. In addition to direct injury, the possibility of contamination cannot be ruled out, and immediate neurosurgical intervention is required to remove bone fragments or foreign matter and to control hemorrhage, edema, and possible infection. A patient with this type of injury is taken directly to the operating room from the emergency department or CAT scanning facility. Postoperatively, the patient is taken directly to the intensive care unit, bypassing the recovery room. This type of patient is gravely ill and the nursing care is extremely demanding, both physically and mentally.

Prior to the admission of the patient to the unit, there must be set up and ready for use a pressure-cycled or volume-cycled ventilator, functional suctioning equipment, several IV poles with volume-regulated infusion pumps, a properly calibrated intracranial monitor, and an arterial line for hemodynamic monitoring. A Swan-Ganz line may also be used for some patients. The nurse who will be responsible for the patient's care is usually notified of the necessary equipment she will need prior to the patient's arrival. After admission to the unit, the patient is attached to the respirator, cardiac monitor, and any other invasive measuring devices, or lines, that may be ordered. The nurse establishes the base-line for vital signs and neurological status before the surgeon leaves the unit. She then examines the patient in a systematic fashion, as in the care of the unconscious patient (described in Chapter 6), and records her findings. The use of diagrams is helpful if the patient has multiple injuries, which is often the case. The patient is placed in bed with at least a thirty-degree elevation of the head. This aids both the reduction of intracranial pressure and thoracic expansion. Initially there will be quite a bit of drainage through the dressing. A waterproof sheet under the head saves a lot of linen changes. Head dressings may be reinforced but not changed by the nurses, at least not in the first few days. If there is no internal intracranial monitoring done on the patient, the nurse will look for the following signs of increased ICP: sudden dilation and fixation of the pupil(s), decreasing and bounding pulse, increasing blood pressure, widening pulse pressure, deceased cardiac output, convulsive activity, and projectile vomiting.

Blood pressure, pulse, respiration, and pupillary checks are made every fifteen minutes initially for the first 24 hours, then every hour thereafter if the patient's condition has stabilized. Fluids are usually limited to 1500 ml per day or less, as there is retention of water and, to a lesser extent, sodium (positive water balance) after cerebral trauma. This positive water balance phase usually lasts from one to three days when it normally corrects itself, although urinary output may be depressed. Fluid intake and diuretic therapy must be carefully considered since water intoxication may occur from overload, thereby increasing cerebral edema. On the other hand, hypovolemia (abnormally low circulating blood volume) must be guarded against. If diuretic therapy is instituted, Mannitol or Urea is the choice of drug for reduction of cerebral edema. However, if the water regulatory center in the brain is damaged and the antidiuretic hormone (ADH) is out of balance, diabetes insipidus develops. This must be treated wtih Pitressin, and serial urine and serum osmolality studies must be done, as well as hourly urinary outputs with specific gravity readings. The specific gravity should not fall below 1.005 or be greater than 1.030, the ideal being 1.010 to 1.020. As for osmolality, the serum should be 280 to 300 milliosmoles/liter (mOsm/liter) and the urine 100 greater than the serum. It may reach as high as 500–800, however. With specific gravity of 1.010, the urine is usually 390. If the patient is suddenly and severely dehydrated, herniation of the brainstem through the foramen magnum may occur.

In addition to monitoring the patient's vital signs and neurological status, maintaining the supporting equipment in good functional order, and meeting fluid, electrolyte, nutritional, and hygiene needs, the nurse must consider the immediate and long-term management of the patient's recovery and return to optimal health. Returning to optimal health may range from total recovery with no neurological deficits in a fully productive individual to spending one's life in a nursing home, totally dependent on others for survival. Even if recovery is possible, the process is a long and arduous one, usually involving extensive rehabilitation. (The subject of rehabilitation is outside the scope of this text.) For the patient, his family, and the nurse, the illness causes a great deal of physical and psychological stress. First, his family learns that their loved one, who is frequently young, has been devastatingly hurt. Even if he lives, the quality of his life is in question. Furthermore, when the family arrives at the hospital, they cannot even recognize their loved one. (It does help to prepare them, prior to admitting them to the unit, for the patient's appearance and his monitoring and treatment equipment.) They need reassurance, but avoid giving false hope. Be honest with them and supportive, and above all, be a friend. They come to rely heavily on the nurse, and it is important that she is mentally strong so she can serve them well.

CLOSED HEAD INJURIES

Injuries of this type include concussions, contusions, lacerations, intracranial hematomas, and skull fractures. Skull fractures may be classified as linear, depressed, or compound.

Concussion is usually defined as a period of unconsciousness due to the transient and reversible disruption of neuronal activity in the reticular formation system of the brainstem. Because anatomic disruption of nerve tissue does not occur as a result of the blow to the head, the neuronal functions return after a period of time, which may range from a few seconds to some minutes. The person sustaining this type of injury should be admitted to the hospital for observation overnight and released the following day if there are no signs of neurological changes.

In *cerebral contusion,* damage to or destruction of nervous tissue has occurred. The area of traumatized tissue may be directly beneath the area of trauma. The basal portion of the brain is one of the most common areas of injury sustained in vehicular collisions, while in the sitting position. In other cases, the injury may be on the opposite side of the blow, in the *countercoup* area. This type is most commonly seen in the temporal and frontal lobes of the brain. This is believed to be the result of the cerebral hemispheres sliding over the sharp, bony protrusions of the sphenoid ridge between the temporal and frontal fossae. In other words, the brain tissue is moving within the cranial vault, striking the rigid skull, then snapping back. This is especially true when there is no skull fracture present. The injury produces an immense amount of pressure or energy (sometimes as high as 30,000 atmospheres), and if this energy is not absorbed by the skull, severe brain injury may occur. This type of injury is referred to as *pulp brain.* Recovery is questionable even though there may not be any apparent external head injuries.

The most severe form of cerebral injury is *cerebral laceration.* A tear in the cerebral tissue breaks the continuity of the tissue as well as disrupting its function. If a vital area of the brain is so injured, the neurological damage is permanent, since the brain tissue does not have the ability to regenerate itself.

Three types of *intracranial hematomas* can result from head injuries: the epidural, the subdural, and the intracerebral hematomas. An *epidural hematoma,* which is often associated with skull fractures, usually results from damage with resultant bleeding from the meningeal arteries. The rapidly expanding hemorrhagic lesion is between the dura and the skull. The pressure produced by the expanding lesion causes distortion and displacement of the brain and compromises vital brainstem functions.

A *subdural hematoma,* on the other hand, is a result of injury to

Head Injuries

the cerebral veins that cross the subdural space leading to the middle sagital sinus. Due to a certain amount of atrophy of brain tissue in the elderly, a subdural hematoma may go undetected for a number of days or even weeks after the injury is sustained and before any clinical manifestations appear.

Intracerebral hematomas result from the rupture of small vascular channels within the brain tissue itself. This type of lesion is produced by the coalescence of hematomas, contused cerebral tissue, and edema. Intracerebral hematomas, or brain lesions, are not limited to the trauma victim, but can be seen in stroke patients as well.

The medical and nursing management of intracranial or intracerebral bleeds includes trephining (burr holes)—boring holes in the skull—to relieve pressure; electric cautery to stop the bleeding; and removal of clots. The nursing care is the same as for any other cerebro-neuro surgery.

MEDICAL MANAGEMENT OF SKULL FRACTURES

Skull fractures are classified as linear, depressed, or compound fractures. Linear fracture is a closed fracture across the bone lengthwise without separation of the two edges, with depressed fracture the bone is pushed inward to press on the brain, and the compound fracture is an open one with splintering of the bone and involvement of the surrounding soft tissue. At times skull fractures can be life saving by disbursing the energy produced by the blow to the head. At other times they may be fatal, especially if the fracture causes a tear in a meningeal artery.

The management of depressed and compound fractures usually consists of craniotomy to elevate the cranial vault and, at times, removal of a bone flap to allow room for the edematous brain tissue to expand. This prevents permanent brain damage, which would otherwise result from prolonged pressure and lack of adequate tissue perfusion of the brain. A large area of the head is shaved for a craniotomy. (Some of the shaved hair should be saved in case the patient's family wishes to buy a wig for the patient to wear during his convalescence.)

CHAPTER 8 | **SPINAL CORD INJURIES**

Spinal cord injuries and fractures result from a variety of forces, such as flexion, hyperextension, and a concomitant rotational movement that results in altered vertebral alignment. If sufficient alteration in the alignment of the vertebral column occurs, rupture of the ligamentous supporting structures results, and the vertebral bodies are either fractured or displaced. The primary concern is not the bony destruction of the spine, however, but the amount of damage that is done to the spinal cord by these displaced or splintered vertebral bodies. The length of time that pressure remains on the spinal cord from dislocations influences the patient's prognosis.

TYPES OF SPINAL CORD LESIONS AND THEIR PHYSIOLOGICAL EFFECTS

Neurological deficits are directly correlated with the level and severity of the spinal injuries and/or the resulting spinal cord lesions (for spinal nerve distribution see dermatomes, Figure 8.1). The mildest form of injury is spinal cord concussion, with transient symptoms and complete recovery. The severest lesion is complete cord transection, resulting in immediate, complete, and irreversible sensory and motor function loss below the level of the injury. The following are typical findings of neurological deficits with complete transverse section injury of the cord at various levels:

At the level of the second and third cervical vertebrae:
1. Complete flaccid body and respiratory paralysis
2. Complete areflexia

Spinal Cord Injuries

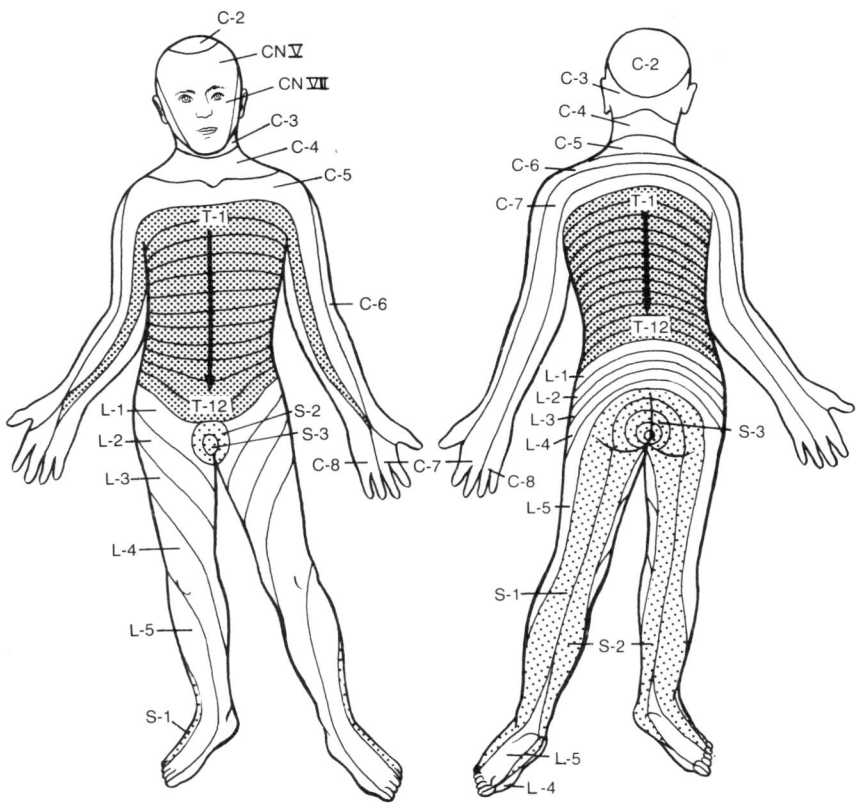

Figure 8.1. Dermatomes—front and back views. Segmental distribution of the spinal nerves to the body's periphery. C–Cervical, T–Thoracic, L–Lumbar, S–Sacral segments.

3. Anesthesia up to the mandible
4. Bowel and bladder retention
5. Death if artificial ventilation is not instituted

At the level of the fifth and sixth cervical vertebrae:

1. Quadriplegia up to the shoulder girdle (some deltoid, pectoral, and bicep functions may be spared, but no intercostal respirations)

2. Complete areflexia (except for some bicep reflex, which may be spared)

3. Anesthesia of the ulnar half of the upper extremities (the outer part of the arms) up to the clavicle

4. Priapism, bowel and bladder retention

At the level of the first through the twelfth thoracic vertebrae:

1. Paraplegia

2. Areflexia of the lower extremities and abdomen, depending on the level of the lesion

3. Anesthesia with a dermatomal distribution—depending on the level of the cord lesion

4. Priapism, bladder and bowel retention

At the level of the first to fifth lumbar vertebrae (cauda equina and conus medullaris):

1. Partial flaccid paraplegia

2. Below the fourth lumbar vertebra, intact abdominal, cremasteric, and patellar tendon reflexes; ankle and plantar reflexes absent

3. Perineal anesthesia and partial or spotty anesthesia of the lower extremities

4. Bowel and bladder retention may or may not be present; if bladder control is lost, it cannot be reestablished.

In addition to complete transverse section of the spinal cord due to direct trauma and its resulting neurological deficits, as described above, there are other types of spinal cord lesions and degrees of neurological deficits or paralysis resulting from them. Examples are the incomplete or partial transection of the cord, the central cord syndrome, and the Brown-Séquard syndrome.

Central cord syndrome pertains to the cervical region of the spinal cord and, as its name suggests, the central portion of the cord is involved. This involvement may be due to hemorrhage, edema, or neoplastic growths. The resulting weakness or paralysis of the upper extremities is disproportionately more than that of the lower extremities.

Incomplete or *partial transection* of the spinal cord on a transverse plane refers to partial division of the spinal cord, resulting in partial paralysis usually ipsilateral in nature, although the patient may have total paralysis initially due to edema and pressure from the sudden volume expansions in the spinal canal. As the edema or blood is reabsorbed and the pressure thereby reduced, sensory and motor function is restored to the contralateral side of the body below the lesion site.

Brown-Séquard syndrome is partial cord transection on a longitudinal axis of the spinal cord. The resulting paralysis and loss of discriminatory sensation to touch, vibration, and position are ipsilateral, but loss of perception of pain and temperature occurs contralaterally in the body below the lesion site.

The two final links of the spinal cord and spinal nerves are the reflex activity and the peripheral nervous system connection. They are responsible for integration and control between all body parts and the central nervous system. The first of these two links is the reflex activity associated with the peripheral nervous system. The loss of these reflexes after injury to the spinal cord is known as spinal shock. Without normal innervation of muscles by the spinal cord segment below the lesion site, flaccid paralysis results. As the edema lessens or the lesion is reduced in size, the spinal shock is resolved and spastic paralysis develops—the activity is purely reflexive in nature. These reflexive activities, however, can be the basis for retraining some of the gross motor functions and movements to useful function by extensive rehabilitation.

The peripheral nervous system extending throughout the body can be divided into specific areas and identified by its supply of spinal nerves. For example, the median, radial, and ulnar nerves of the upper extremities form the connection between the periphery and the sixth, seventh, and eighth cervical spinal nerves and the first thoracic spinal nerve. The sciatic and femoral nerves innervating the lower extremities connect with the second, third, fourth, and fifth lumbar nerves. If paralysis occurs in either area, the suspected lesion site can be clearly identified.

The skin's innervation also corresponds to spinal cord segments, connecting with a specific skin area called a dermatome. Knowledge of the dermatomal distribution is a highly useful assessment parameter and is necessary for accurate localization of the level of the spinal cord lesion (for detailed charts on dermatomes, see Figure 8.1).

Whether the pathology is expressed as edema, hemorrhage, direct trauma, inflammation, infection of the spinal meninges, or neoplastic growths within the spinal canal or the cord, its underlying cause and duration determine the symptoms the patient will be exhibiting and how successful the recovery will be. If the lesion develops suddenly, as in the case of acute trauma, and transection apparently is complete, the resulting flaccid paralysis will change to spastic paralysis (these are only some jerking movements) within a few weeks. In this case the patient and his family must be told what to expect so that they do not interpret the spastic activity in the limbs as an indication that complete recovery may occur. As stated earlier, some reflexic activities may be retrained, but fine motor coordination cannot be achieved. If the spinal cord lesion develops slowly, however, as in the case of a neoplastic growth, and the pressure on the cord is gradual, the resulting paralysis will be spastic and become flaccid from the evolving tumor mass until complete transection of the cord occurs. This, of course, alerts the care provider to the fact that the patient's condition is deteriorating, and nursing care plans will be modified to reflect the patient's progressive disability.

EVALUATION AND MANAGEMENT OF SPINAL INJURIES

Every patient presenting in the emergency department with a history of significant trauma associated with motor vehicular collision, diving mishap, fall from heights, or contact sports must be considered and handled as a spinal-injured victim until careful evaluation and radiological studies prove otherwise. The spine must therefore be kept straight and immobile. The victim should be placed on a rigid surface, such as a spine or fracture board. If a board is not available, the door of an automobile or the ground may be used until qualified help arrives with proper equipment. The neck is stabilized with a soft cervical collar or a rolled up towel. If neither is available, keeping the patient from turning his head from side to side will accomplish the same thing. This is often difficult as the patient may have been drinking, he may be frightened and in pain, or he may need to vomit. The fear of possible back injury and paralysis will prompt him to move or try to sit up. He may become extremely unreasonable and demanding in his behavior. Such a patient will usually voice a fear of paralysis and, most often, complain of severe pain in the neck or back. If the lesion is in the lower cervical and upper thoracic region, the patient will complain of severe pain in the neck, shoulders, and one or both arms. The patient must be kept still on the spine board until he is transferred to the appropriate bed—a regular hospital bed with a bed board, a Stryker frame and skeletal traction, a circo-electric bed, or a kinetic bed. It is not advisable to transfer the patient more than once from the time he is picked up at the scene of his injury until he is placed in his hospital bed. It takes at least five persons to effect his transfer safely. Under no circumstances should the patient be removed from the spinal board for radiographic (X-rays) studies—he should be X-rayed while lying on the spinal board. The cervical collar should remain in place at all times. If it needs to be taken off for X-rays, the emergency department physician is the only person to do so. *Under no circumstances, at any time, or in any situation, is the nurse or X-ray technician permitted to remove the collar.* If the physician removes the collar, he must maintain gentle traction on the neck by grasping the patient on the mandibular angles of the jaw to keep him from bending his neck forward or turning his head from side to side, and being careful not to apply too much traction, which may cause hyperflexion of the cervical spine and increase spinal cord damage.

Both the emergency department physician and the nurse must be aware of the possibility of added spinal cord damage and the devastating sequelae that may result from injudicious handling of the patient with injuries of this type. It is their responsibility to protect the patient from further injury or damage. The emergency department physician must accompany the patient to the radiology department to supervise any necessary changes in the patient's position, and remain with the patient until satisfactory views of the spine have been obtained and developed. Cross-table lateral films of the neck, using an upright Bucky or grid cassette, should be obtained first to rule out major fractures or dislocations of the upper cervical spine. The lower cervical and upper thoracic spine is very hard to visualize. Sometimes several X-rays are required, and even then some fractures may be missed. A laminagraphy may be necessary to establish correct diagnosis of fractures or dislocations of the lower cervical spine, particularly those involving the odontoid process. Fractures with severe cord compression or transection above the third cervical vertebra are usually not compatible with life due to the loss of phrenic nerve function. If the patient has to be turned for X-rays of the thoracic, lumbar, and lumbosacral spine, he must be turned by two persons in log fashion to keep the spine in proper alignment. (In log rolling, a turn sheet or blanket is very helpful.) Spot views of the area of local tenderness and pain should be taken in these longer segments of the spine.

The systemic approach to spinal X-ray evaluation by the "ABC" method is briefly described below:

Alignment is assessed by comparing the height of the anterior and posterior margins of the vertebral bodies. These are almost equal in adults and older children. If not, the vertebral body has a wedge-shaped appearance, which is usually indicative of a compression fracture.

Bony mineralization assessment is important to establish preexisting disease, such as osteoporosis or osteomalacia. Demineralization, however, may indicate subluxation of the atlas and axis or the other cervical vertebrae (common in rheumatoid arthritis). As much as 2.5 mm of space may separate the anterior ring of the atlas from the odontoid process. If there is no history of a preexisting spinal condition, the radiolucent linear or comminuted sharp lines indicate probable fractures of the lamina peducles or neuronal arches. On the other hand, localized radiodensity is indicative of compression fracture.

Cartilage space assessment is done to evaluate the supportive soft tissue's integrity. If traumatic disruption of the soft tissue is present, subluxation or dislocation must be considered. This type of injury renders the cervical spine extremely unstable.

The condition of *soft tissue* must be evaluated. Careful observation is given to changes in height of the intervertebral disc spaces, which are decreased in degenerative conditions. Areas to be assessed most carefully are those between the fifth and sixth cervical, and from the fourth lumbar to the first sacral vertebral discs. These spaces receive the greatest pivotal and mechanical load. Observing the soft tissue space anterior to the cervical spine will aid in detecting fractures. If the retropharyngeal space anterior to the third cervical vertebra is greater than 5 mm, edema or hemorrhage is present in that area of the spinal cord. The thoracic and lumbar vertebrae are quite stable from dislocations, but wedge fractures (a wedge-shaped piece of the vertebral body breaks off and is pressing on the spinal cord) are common, and decompression may be necessary. At this point, the emergency department physician turns the patient's care over to a competent surgeon or neurosurgeon. He will perform a decompressive procedure or a laminectomy to relieve the pressure. If a spinal fusion is also necessary, it will be deferred to a later date when the edema from the trauma has subsided, after decompression. A myelogram is usually done prior to surgery for assessment of the location and size of the lesion.

Stabilization of spinal fractures is accomplished through several different types of skeletal tractions, with Crutchfield tongs the most common type used for C-spine fractures. By drilling shallow holes in the skull above the ears, the pins are inserted and the half-circle metal ring attached. In the center of the half-circle is a rope pulley that holds the weight and provides the traction. The weight (eight to ten pounds is usually used) must hang free to maintain traction. This type of traction can be used on the Stryker frame, circo-electric bed, or kinetic treatment table. If the patient is in a regular hospital bed, he may have a Philadelphia collar (four-poster bar) traction, or a halo traction, which allows him mobility, but if he is placed in a spica (body cast), this again immobilizes the patient. The latter type of traction is not used on a paralyzed patient, who must be nursed on one or the other of the neuro-ortho beds.

The neurotrauma patient needs special or additional care beyond the routine nursing care that each hospitalized patient receives. This additional care is specific to neurotrauma patients because their special needs are both acute and long term. Also, since recovery of normal function is questionable and most neurotrauma patients fall into the young age group, the situation is difficult for both the patient and the nurse. It is extremely hard to keep up the patient's morale when he faces possible permanent loss of function.

NURSING MANAGEMENT OF THE PATIENT WITH SPINAL CORD INJURY OR LESIONS

It takes a special nurse to do a special job. He or she needs to be in good physical health and possess emotional stability along with plenty of empathy. The empathy displayed by a kind word, soft touch, or reassuring countenance goes a long way in keeping up the patient's morale. Compassion and emotions should not be permitted to interfere with good judgment and logic, however. The nurse who does not possess strong emotional stability or who becomes too deeply involved with the patient may be unable to render necessary or good care. Along with being emotionally strong, she needs to possess both native intelligence and an innate curiosity.

Ventilation, Circulation, Elimination, and Assimilation

After the patient has been stabilized in the emergency department and transferred to the ICU, four major considerations become foremost in the nurse's mind. A plan must be formulated to meet the patient's needs for ventilation, circulation, elimination, and assimilation. Ventilation and circulation may have been stabilized in the emergency room, as they are the primary considerations in preserving vital functions. After a thorough evaluation of the adequacy of ventilation and circulation, the nurse will consider elimination and assimilation.

Often the spinal-injured patient is paralyzed, temporarily or permanently, and an indwelling catheter is necessary to manage urinary output. This is especially true if the patient has been given, or is to get, Decadron and Mannitol on admission to the unit. They both will act as diuretics. He may be nauseated or vomiting and need gastric decompression right away, as he cannot tilt his head to the side to avoid aspiration of vomitus. If the patient is turned, at least two nurses are required if he is on a neuro-ortho bed, four when he is nursed in a regular bed. Nurses who work with neuro-ortho beds need to have a good knowledge of their function.

Assimilation is not an immediate consideration, but a care plan should at least be started for nutritional management. Unless the patient has sustained cerebral injuries, he will be awake and alert, but feeding him orally should not commence for about a week, especially for quadriplegics. The shock their body has received takes at least three days to dissipate, and nausea and vomiting often result from solid foods. Since their nutritional needs must be met for healing and to avoid a stress (peptic) ulcer, tube feedings of Vivonex or Ensure in small amounts are started as soon as the patient has bowel sounds.

A high protein, high vitamin, high caloric intake will aid in healing and prevention of pressure sores. Fluids, unless contraindicated, must be given at a level of at least 3000 ml in 24 hours. Since good nutrition alone cannot prevent the occurrence of pressure sores, the patient's position must be changed every two hours and meticulous skin care given. The most important component of skin care is keeping it clean and dry at all times.

Each time the patient is turned, his neurological status should be noted. This is to establish any change in sensation or motor function. If there is any deterioration in either, the physician must be notified immediately. He must have accurate details of the status change and, of course, it must be correctly documented.

Intake and Output

Accurate intake and output records are mandatory. The urine should be checked for sugar and acetone, amount, color, odor, acidity (pH), and specific gravity. The two most common complications following injury are urinary tract infections and static pneumonia. Particular attention must therefore be paid to the urine and its characteristics. The management of defecation is accomplished by prevention of constipation. But if it occurs, suppositories or enemas every two to three days are given. Neither quadriplegics nor paraplegics have bowel control.

Medication

In neurotrauma nursing, medications are all given symptomatically, to maintain the patient's comfort and morale and to prevent or treat complications as they arise. Meeting the patient's physical needs is not enough, however, and to attend the body but ignore the (soul) psyche would be a grave error.

Emotional Needs

The morale of the patient has a great deal to do with his ability to recover and to deal realistically with his limitations. To maintain the patient's morale at all times is much more difficult than to ensure safety and comfort. The health care providers, particularly the nurses who are in constant attendance on the patient, must not only possess good mental health or emotional strength. They must also be honest and have a great deal of understanding and empathy. The young adult patient may ask about his chances of full recovery. He may already know his prognosis but may be unable to accept it. The nurse must deal with his questions honestly, regardless of how unpleasant the answers may be. Often recovery cannot be predicted, and the nurse should say so. If there is residual function left in the patient's limbs, abilities rather than disabilities should be stressed.

If the patient becomes angry and abusive, the nurse must remain pleasant—firm but caring at all times. To avoid withdrawal or deep depression, every effort should be made to keep the patient pleasantly or constructively occupied—for example, listening to the radio, watching television, or reading. Special mirrors can be mounted onto the neuro-ortho beds that enable the patient to watch television. The same frame is suitable for holding a book. If the patient is a quadriplegic, he may read when he is on his abdomen and the nurse only has to turn the pages for him. While the patient is in the prone position, the nurse can brush his teeth also—patients seem to prefer brushing to having suction used for oral care.

Friends and relatives are to be encouraged to visit. Specific times should be set aside for visitors when nursing functions will not interfere with the visiting period and vice versa. Interestingly enough, after the initial news of the patient's accident, there are literally dozens of visitors demanding to see the patient, but as time goes on, they slowly dwindle to very few in number. This should be prevented, if at all possible, by asking visitors to space their visits and limit their numbers, or take turns in coming to visit. As this is an extended type of illness that may go on for weeks or months, they all will have their chance to come and cheer up the patient. On the other hand, stress the importance of their return. Initially, the visitation time limit should be brief and visitors limited to family. This is to ensure proper rest periods for the patient. Proper rest is as important to the healing process and maintenance of morale as nutrition. As the patient recovers, his visitation periods should be extended and the number of visitors may be increased, especially in the case of close friends or schoolmates. In the case of a young parent, his or her children may be allowed to visit. This decision, however, must be left up to the family. The author believes that seeing the parent incapacitated is less traumatizing psychologically to the child than the imagined abandonment he is likely to experience when the parent does not return home. In any case the patient should be involved with as many people as is safely possible.

CHAPTER 9 | ACUTE MEDICAL-NEUROLOGIC CONDITIONS

A number of medical-neurologic conditions, in addition to the ones previously mentioned, require nursing management in the intensive care setting because they may be life threatening. These conditions include: cerebrovascular accidents (CVA) or stroke, cerebral thrombosis, cerebral embolism, subarachnoid hemorrhage (SAH), meningitis, encephalitis, poliomyelitis, Guillain-Barré syndrome, tetanus, and myasthenia gravis crisis.

The two major cerebral bleeding disorders are *cerebrovascular accidents (CVA)* and *subarachnoid hemorrhage (SAH)*. Perhaps "stroke" is a more appropriate term to describe cerebrovascular bleeding, since it is not an accident in the usual sense. The underlying pathological process usually originates outside the cranium and may not even be the direct outcome of vascular problems. Therefore the term "stroke" will be used here.

STROKES AND HYPERTENSION

Stroke is a major health problem in the United States. Approximately 100,000 persons die each year from cerebral bleeds, cerebral thrombotic, or embolitic events, and another 100,000 are left with various functional and/or cognitive neurological deficits as a result of it. The age group most commonly affected are persons from the fifties and upward; however, younger adults have suffered from strokes, too. The younger age group is more susceptible to strokes if they are obese or have a history of hypertension, coronary vascular disease, or diabetes mellitus; or if they are women who use oral contraceptives.

Although there are a number of causes for strokes, the leading cause is hypertension, which is, to some extent, a preventable health problem. Hypertension can, in many instances, be prevented or minimized if the public is aware of and complies with guidelines for controlling it. These guidelines include dietary habit modification, such as the avoidance of excessive sugar, salt, and high cholesterol intake. Excessive consumption of alcoholic beverages and the use of tobacco should also be avoided. It is important to exercise regularly and to minimize stress if possible, and when it is not, to learn to deal with stress more effectively. These factors all contribute to blood pressure control.

There are four terms to describe hypertension: essential or primary, secondary, malignant, and labile.

In *essential hypertension,* the most prevalent type, the diastolic blood pressure is the best indicator of the severity of the disease. If the systolic pressure rises, it is usually secondary to the diastolic elevation. The American Medical Association classifies hypertension as follows: A diastolic blood pressure of 90 to 120 mm Hg is mild hypertension; moderate hypertension is a diastolic pressure of 120 to 140 mm Hg, and diastolic pressure above 140 mm Hg is severe hypertension. Although a healthier life style and eating habits aid in the control of essential hypertension, its exact cause is not known. The five hemodynamic conditions affected by prolonged hypertension are cardiac output, blood volume, arterial wall elastance, peripheral vascular resistance, and the blood's viscosity. These hemodynamic functions are influenced by the nervous, cardiac, endocrine (hormonal), and renal systems. In turn, sustained elevated blood pressure causes atherosclerotic changes in the brain, retina of the eyes, heart, and the kidneys. If this cycle continues over an extended period of time, significant vascular changes occur.

Although the underlying pathology of cerebral thrombosis and embolism differs from cerebral hemorrhage in that they block the cerebral vessels and thereby deprive the brain from its necessary circulation and nutrients, the clinical presentation is much the same in all strokes. The differentiation in diagnosis and the prognosis are based on the speed of occurrence of the stroke and the patient's past medical history. The stroke due to cerebral thrombosis is slow in its evolution. It is not activity-related and may be preceded by focal neurological deficits, complaints of headache and vertigo, and seizure activity followed by loss of consciousness. Stroke due to an embolism is also not activity-related, but its evolution is rapid as a blood clot or plaque can reach the brain within seconds from its original site. Very seldom does the patient have time to complain of a headache before he loses consciousness. A stroke resulting from cerebral hemorrhage develops rapidly. It is activity-related, and it is preceded by severe headache and minor focal neurological symptoms before loss of consciousness occurs. The level of coma will depend on the extent of interruption of blood supply to the brain and/or the amount of increase in intracranial volume and intracranial pressure. On recovering consciousness from a hemorrhagic stroke, the patient has contralateral hemiplegia and may have speech disturbances or aphasia, depending on the site of the bleed or the hemisphere in which the lesion occurred. The affected side is spastic. Other common signs of a cerebral hemorrhage include nuchal rigidity (a sign of meningeal irritation), hyperreflexic tendons, and generalized convulsions.

ASSESSMENT AND MANAGEMENT OF PATIENTS WITH STROKES

To have a clear and complete picture on which to base diagnosis and modality of treatment, a thorough medical history, physical examination, neurological assessment, and adjunct laboratory and special diagnostic studies must be performed. When taking the patient's previous medical history, the health care provider must include the following questions:

1. Preexisting medical conditions—does the patient suffer from conditions such as diabetes mellitus, coronary vascular disease, or transient ischemic attacks (TIAs)?

2. Precipitating factors—what type of activity was the patient engaged in at the time of the onset of symptoms, and what was their mode of onset?

3. Has the patient been on anticoagulant therapy, and if so, on what drug, how much, and for how long?

Next the care provider should carry out a thorough physical assessment. This may be done by another nurse due to the urgency of the patient's clinical condition at the time of admission, which should be the first consideration in all cases. The physical assessment should include blood pressure readings from both arms, auscultation and palpation of all major arterial courses such as the carotid, vertebral, and subclavian arteries. The apical pulse should be counted for a full minute. Any cardiac irregularities, thrills, or bruits noted in arteries must be brought to the physician's attention. Thrills and bruits are suggestive of obstructive events—that is, partial or total occlusion of the artery by plaque deposits, blood clots, or vegetative bacterial clumps such as those found in bacterial endocarditis, which may break away and occlude one of the carotid arteries. Blood flow through a narrowed vessel will be expressed by bruits, whereas a thrill is a result of complete occlusion of the artery and reversal of blood flow, which cannot pass the obstruction. All examinations are to be done bilaterally for comparative data. Thermographic examination of the skin above the obstruction will prove it to be much cooler than below the site. The temperature difference is a good indicator of the degree of obstruction. Doppler scan is performed to establish the carotid artery's efficiency. An ophthalmic examination is made to evaluate the pupils, the optic discs, and the retinal arteries, which are indicators of increased intracranial pressure. In addition, an electrocardiogram (ECG), radiographic studies of the chest and skull, an electroencephalogram (EEG), brain scanning with radioisotopes, a computer-assisted tomography (CAT scan), cerebral angiography, a spinal tap, and various blood studies are performed.

X-ray studies are done to exclude occult head and chest injuries. Brain scanning establishes the site of the lesion but cannot differentiate it. An electroencephalogram will locate the site of lesion, as the brain waves in this area will be slow or flat; however, it supplies information relating only to the surface of the brain and cannot reflect pontine or medullary lesions. Cerebral angiography establishes the cerebral blood flow status. The CAT scan is capable of diagnosing the site, size, and depth of the lesion, while a spinal tap differentiates thrombotic and embolitic strokes from hemorrhagic strokes. The spinal fluid with hemorrhagic strokes is bloody, whereas with thrombotic and embolitic strokes it is clear. The spinal fluid pressure is elevated (greater than 180 mm Hg) in all strokes.

The nursing and medical management of the stroke patient is

symptomatic. The focus is on stabilizing the blood pressure, supporting vital functions, reducing the intracranial pressure, and preventing or controlling seizure activity (see Chapter 6, the care of the unconscious and seizuring patient).

SUBARACHNOID HEMORRHAGE

Subarachnoid hemorrhage can result from trauma, aneurysm of cerebral arteries, and arteriovenous malformation. The latter two are usually a result of congenital weakness of the arterial wall and arteriovenous shunts, respectively. The preexisting weakness in the artery cannot take the added stress that results from arteriosclerotic changes, systemic infections, stressful living situations, and ruptures. The most common sites are the arteries in the occipital lobe. Blood replaces the cerebrospinal fluid circulating in the subarachnoid space, and neurological signs and symptoms will be present. The size of the bleed determines the severity of the neurological symptoms and/or deficits the patient will have. A leaking aneurysm will cause mild symptoms such as headache, nuchal rigidity, visual disturbances, irritability, restlessness, photophobia, and positive Kernig's and Brudzinski's signs. It can occur at rest, with physical activity, or from emotional stress. The first sign of a bleed is a severe headache. If massive hemorrhage occurs and the ventricles fill up with blood, the patient's condition rapidly deteriorates to coma and death.

As with any cerebral bleed, previous medical history, a complete physical examination, and neurological evaluation are done. Supportive care is instituted as necessary, and the treatment is symptomatic. Two specific studies are performed to confirm the presence and extent of subarachnoid hemorrhage—a spinal tap and a cerebral arteriogram or angiography. Both must be carried out with utmost care and constant monitoring of the patient. With a spinal tap the release of some of the built-up pressure can cause structural changes or brain shifting and brain herniation. The dye injected with the angiographic studies may cause severe vasospasms, depriving the brain of adequate cerebral circulation, and death may result. Life support equipment must be at hand, and if the patient's condition deteriorates, the procedure should be aborted. Angiograms are done the first day to establish the severity of the hemorrhage. If it is mild to moderate, surgical intervention is considered to repair the damaged vessel. If the hemorrhage is severe, however, a more conservative approach to medical management is instituted, aimed at the reduction of increased intracranial pressure and maintenance of the systemic pressure to preserve the necessary cerebral perfusion pressure. Absolute bedrest, sedatives, anticonvulsants, and the intravenous administration of Amicar (aminocaproic acid) are required. Amicar is used to prevent further or recurrent bleeding by eliminating fibrinolytic activity within the cerebrospinal fluid and to inhibit clot lysis systematically.

POLIOMYELITIS

Poliomyelitis is an acute viral infection affecting the anterior horn cells of the spinal cord, the motor cells of the brainstem, and other parts of the brain. It is categorized according to the types of cells affected—bulbar, encephalitic, and spinal. The symptoms of spinal cord involvement include weakness or paralysis of the muscles in the trunk and extremities. If the higher centers in the brain are involved, the symptoms will include headache, drowsiness, hyperthermia, and mental confusion, and unconsciousness may occur. If the brainstem is involved, the patient will experience difficulty with swallowing and respiration. Oropharyngeal suctioning and respiratory assistance may become necessary. A spinal tap will reveal a high white blood count (WBC) and elevated protein (greater than 45 mg / 100 ml) levels.

Nursing care is done under *strict isolation*. It is symptomatic and palliative, with prevention of complications as its main focus. People infected with polio virus are rarely seen today since the introduction of the injectible Salk vaccine in 1955 and the oral vaccine by Sabin in 1958. If it does occur, it is due to lack of proper immunization of children. Both vaccine preparations are freely obtainable at public health departments and health clinics in major cities. The American Academy of Pediatrics recommends the initial administration of oral Sabine vaccine to every child at the age of two months.

ENCEPHALITIS

Encephalitis or "sleeping sickness" is an infection of the brain caused by various strains of viruses. These viruses include eastern and western equine encephalitis (a primary viral infection of birds transmitted to horses and man by mosquitoes), herpes simplex, herpes zoster, rabies, poliomyelitis, and echo. It may also result as a complication from both types of measles, from chicken pox, mumps, and as a post-vaccination reaction to rabies, yellow fever, and pertussis vaccines.

These viral infections cause diffuse damage to the nerve cells in the brain and the brain's vascular system. The proliferation of glial cells increases cerebral volume and, thereby, intracranial pressure. The onset of the infection may be insidious or sudden, with symptoms of increased intracranial pressure and hyperpyrexia. If left untreated it may progress from lethargy to coma and death. Even past the acute phase of the disease, the comatose state of the patient may last from weeks to months. As a result, the popular lay term for encephalitis is "sleeping sickness." Although death may occur from the disease, most patients recover with proper treatment.

Medical and nursing management of the patient with encephalitis is supportive, symptomatic, and preventive. Hypertonic solutions intraveneously, steroids, and cerebral dehydrators are used to reduce or minimize the effects of cerebral edema. Mechanical ventilation will usually be accomplished via tracheostomy, since an endotracheal tube left in place longer than seven days may result in laryngeal necrosis and attrition. The patient is placed in strict isolation from one to three weeks or until the immunological viral studies (of the patient's blood serum and cerebrospinal fluid) establish the causative agent of the disease.

During the recovery phase the patient's sleeping pattern is reversed. Attempts should be made to keep the patient awake during the daytime hours, and a mild sedative should be given at night to aid sleep. As a result of the diffused and prolonged brain infection, the patient may suffer from various functional disabilities requiring long-term care and rehabilitation. Post-encephalitic seizures are common, and the patient may require anticonvulsive medication. He must be taught the importance of taking his medication and keeping appointments for follow-up visits to his physician. During these office visits, serial electroencephalograms are done for reevaluation of brain wave activity. At least one person living with the patient should be instructed concerning his medication and his activity limits, since the patient may also have cognitive disorders. Home health care may be necessary after discharge from the hospital or rehabilitation facility.

MENINGITIS

Meningitis is an acute inflammation of the pia mater (inner layer) and the arachnoid membrane (middle layer) of the brain and/or covering of the spinal cord secondary to systemic bacterial, viral, protozoal, or fungal infections. Meningitis may follow septicemia from localized infections, including those involving (a) the head, (b) upper respiratory tract, (c) infections of the oronasal pharynx, the middle ear (otitis media), tonsils, mastoid process, or the eyes, (d) lower respiratory (lung) infections, and (e) infections of the bones and heart valves (bacterial endocarditis). It may also result from a ruptured brain abcess or open skull fracture.

Patients with bacterial meningitis will experience all the signs and symptoms of infection—chills, fever, and elevated white blood cell count (WBC). With viral infection, the temperature is usually normal and the meningeal irritation is expressed by headaches, irritability, and stiffness in the neck and back. In severe cases the patient may assume an opisthotonus position—hyperdorsiflexion of the neck and spine. The patient is checked for Brudzinski's and Kernig's signs to evaluate the presence and the degree of meningeal involvement. Brudzinski's sign is said to be positive if the patient cannot tolerate forward neck flexion onto the chest while in the dorsal recumbent position, due to severe pain. The Kernig's sign is said to be positive if pain or resistance is encountered when the patient is required to straighten the knees from a supine (flat on back) position with the hips and knees flexed. This maneuver is specific to spinal meningeal inflammation. A spinal tap is performed to confirm the diagnosis of meningitis and to identify the causative agent (for details of CSF pressure and analysis, see

Chapter 3). Antibiotic therapy, however, is generally instituted before laboratory findings are completed. Drugs usually given are Penicillin-G, Ampicillin, Kanamycin, or Gentamycin. In addition to antibiotic therapy, the patient is given anticonvulsants to prevent or control seizures and medication to reduce cerebral edema. As with other types of neurological patients, nursing care is symptomatic and supportive.

TETANUS (LOCKJAW)

Tetanus is an acute infectious disease process caused by the toxins of the anaerobic, spore-forming *Clostridium tetani bacillus*. It is contracted through open wounds, usually of the deep puncture type, from the soil. The onset of symptoms may take up to three weeks after the infective organism is introduced into the body. The symptoms include involvement of the jaw muscles and difficulty in opening the mouth. As the toxins travel up the spinal cord to the brain, particularly to the medulla oblongata, the symptoms become more severe due to minute hemorrhages, edema, and inflammation in the medulla. The progression of the disease brings about headache, neck and back pain, stiffness of the muscles of the back and neck, and, in some cases, the assumption of an opisthotonus position. Pharyngolaryngeal spasms make swallowing and breathing difficult, if not impossible. The classical facial expression of the patient with tetanus is a tense and immobile face, with wrinkled forehead and the corners of the mouth drawn with the lips pouting in a fixed, ghastly smile (risus sardonicus). The deep tendons are hyperreflexic, and the slightest stimulation can increase pain and spasms in the affected muscles, resulting in convulsive activity. The patient's temperature and pulse are both elevated.

With routine active immunization through tetanus vaccine, given with diphtheria and pertussis vaccine in early childhood, the incidence of tetanus is relatively low in the United States. Routine booster injections for tetanus are to be given every ten years to injury-free individuals, and every five years if any injury occurs that makes the person susceptible to tetanus. The management of the patient with tetanus will depend largely on past active immunization. The patient who has had active immunization against the disease will require a booster injection of tetanus toxoid; if not, he will be given a large dose of tetanus antitoxoid intravenously, or a complete series of active immunizations with tetanus toxoid. *An important caution:* if the patient has a history of sensitivity to horse serum, he is to be given (human) tetanus immunoglobulin (intramuscularly, not intravenously) instead of the tetanus antitoxin. Large doses of Penicillin are also given intramuscularly. The site of the injury should be meticulously cleansed with germicidal solution, the wound debrided, surgically scraped out and cauterized, and left open to air. A whirlpool treatment, with betadine added to the water, once or twice a day may be helpful.

As the patient is extremely sensitive to any type of stimuli, which may produce seizure activity, he should be nursed in a quiet, semidark room. As a rule he is heavily sedated and must be closely monitored for swallowing and respiratory difficulties. A tracheostomy and mechanical ventilation are often required for several weeks. The choice of sedative (tranquilizer) is Thorazine for its effectiveness in relieving reflex muscle spasms. *An important caution: the usual ice packs or iced-water and alcohol baths as cooling measures for reduction of high temperatures are to be avoided with the tetanus patient.* These measures may trigger extremely severe muscle spasms that may result in fractures of long bones.

The morbidity and mortality rate for tetanus patients depends, in part, on the prompt administration of the correct antidote, prevention of complications, and good nursing care. The patient's fluid and nutritional needs are met by naso-gastric feedings, and elimination is managed with an indwelling urinary catheter and bowel evacuation by administering stool softeners or cathartics. The use of rectal suppositories or colon lavages is not permitted, as they may trigger seizures. In addition to the above treatment, the prevention and treatment of increased intracranial pressure are incorporated into the patient's care. Even with the best possible medical and nursing management, the mortality rate of patients infected with tetanus is 30 to 40 percent.

GUILLAIN-BARRÉ SYNDROME

Guillain-Barré syndrome, an acute polineuritis involving the motor components of the spinal and cranial motor nerve roots, is probably caused by a virus. In the early stages of the disease it may be mistaken for influenza. The onset of symptoms is acute and includes headache, hyperpyrexia, aching limbs, and general malaise. As the disease progresses, severe pain, weakness, and paralysis of individual muscle groups occur, starting with the fingers and toes and spreading upward to the chest, neck, and face. It spreads up to and includes the vital centers in the medulla oblongata. While there is no sensory loss, the loss of motor nerve control may culminate in death due to respiratory arrest if the patient goes untreated. The primary focus of care, therefore, is on ventilatory assistance and oropharyngeal suctioning. The patient cannot speak, swallow, or breathe due to the paralysis of the seventh, ninth, and tenth cranial nerves resulting from the medullary involvement. Depending on the degree of involvement of the lost motor functions, recovery may start within a few days, but full recovery may take up to eighteen months.

The diagnosis of Guillain-Barré syndrome is based on the patient's history, physical assessment findings, and the cerebrospinal fluid analysis. The cerebrospinal fluid will show a slightly elevated white blood cell count of 10–50 cells/mm^3 (norm 9–5 cells/mm^3). The protein levels are extremely high, sometimes reaching 600–800 mgs/100 ml (norm 15–45 mgs/100 ml).

As with other infectious neurological diseases, the medical and nursing management of the patient with Guillain-Barré syndrome is symptomatic, palliative, and preventive in nature. Correct posturing of the patient with Guillain-Barré syndrome is the same as for the patient with serious cervical spinal cord injury, except that skeletal traction is not applied. The patient needs to be turned by two persons every two hours, given meticulous skin care, and correctly positioned when on his sides to avoid foot and/or wrist drop. His nutritional needs should be met by naso-gastric feeding, although total parenteral nutrition may be instituted the first seven to ten days of his hospitalization (for details see Chapter 8 on care of the spinal cord–injured patient).

MYASTHENIA GRAVIS

Myasthenia gravis is not an infectious disease process but a progressively debilitating neuromuscular disorder. Because of its progressively debilitating nature, the patient with myasthenia gravis will be cared for in the intensive care unit, especially in the case of myasthenia gravis crisis. During the crisis period the patient's oropharyngeal and respiratory muscles are so weak that he cannot manage his normal oral and pulmonary secretions or maintain a sufficient pulmonary vital capacity. The patient's condition during crisis warrants a tracheostomy and ventilatory support with a positive pressure-cycled or volume ventilator.

The exact underlying pathology of myasthenia gravis is not known, but several theories have been offered: it may be caused by (a) an acetylocholine production deficiency, (b) an end-plate disorder at the neuromuscular junction, or (c) some type of disorder within the muscle fibers themselves. However, there is increasing evidence that the thymus gland plays an important role in the body's immunological process, and it has been suggested that myasthenia gravis is produced by an autoimmune mechanism that in some way destroys or inactivates the neuromuscular junction. The last of these proposals led to the belief that if a thymectomy were performed, the patient's condition would markedly improve or be completely cured. This operation has been proved effective in about 80 to 90 percent of the cases, especially in female patients under thirty-five years of age. Because the incidence of myasthenia gravis is highest in women between the ages of fifteen and fifty years, this treatment represents an important advance.

Diagnosis of myasthenia gravis is based on the following:

1. *The patient's history or chief complaints,* which include progressive muscular weakness expressed by the inability to chew or swallow, difficulty in voice production and breathing, maintaining the eyelids open, and finally, general exhaustion. The patient revives with rest, but as the disease advances, the patient's strength does not return, even with rest. Although the patient may not be able to move his muscles, there is no evidence of central or peripheral nervous system involvement with muscular atrophy or loss of sensation, and the apparent muscular paralysis is transitory.

2. *The current physical findings* include a blank, expressionless face; ptosis (drooping) of the upper eyelids, with the head tilted back to facilitate vision; inability to chew or swallow, with frequent nasal regurgitation of oral fluids; inaudible or nasal voice;

and difficulty with or the inability to maintain adequate ventilation.

3. *Confirmation of the diagnosis* is obtained by administration of Tensilon 2 mg intravenously. If there is no response to the initial dose within 30 seconds, another 8 mg is given over a one-minute period. Tensilon is especially useful in evaluating the degree of weakness of the oropharyngeal and ocular muscles, and the patient shows spontaneous improvement. Its disadvantage is that its effects only last about five minutes. Prostigmin, the other test drug, is given intramuscularly in a dose of 1.5 to 2 mg. It takes up to an hour for its clinical effect to occur, but it lasts up to several hours. It is most beneficial in the evaluation of motor function of the extremities.

After the diagnosis is confirmed and the patient's condition stabilized, the focus is on patient education. The patient must be made to understand that there is no positive medical cure for myasthenia gravis, but that with proper care and treatment it is possible to remain a highly productive member of society for many years after the initial diagnosis, and that motherhood can be successfully achieved. Furthermore, the nurse must stress the importance of avoiding upper respiratory infections, excessive fatigue, extreme emotional stress, smoking, drinking, prolonged exposure to the sun, or extremely cold temperature. Also to be avoided are medications that contain opiate derivatives, curare, procainamide, quinidine, quinine, magnesium sulfate, or chlorpromazine. General anesthesia should not be given. A proper well-balanced diet and adequate rest are important, as is taking prescribed medications such as Mestinon, Prostigmin, or Mytelase. The patient should carry a type-written card containing the above medical information.

CHAPTER 10 | NEUROLOGICAL DIAGNOSTIC STUDIES

In addition to a complete medical history, physical examination, and various laboratory studies, a thorough neurological assessment is made at the time of admission. However, to establish a definitive neurological diagnosis, evaluate the extent of the neurological damage, and formulate a plan for the correct treatment modality, specific neurological studies are necessary. The following are the most commonly performed neurological diagnostic studies:

1. Electroencephalogram
2. Echoencephalography
3. Pneumoencephalogram
4. Spinal tap or lumbar puncture
5. Noninvasive radiographic studies of the skull and spine
6. Cerebral angiography
7. Ventriculography
8. Myelography
9. Isotope brain scanning
10. Computer-assisted tomography
11. Caloric test for vestibular function
12. Glucose tolerance test
13. Iodine sweat test.

THE ELECTROENCEPHALOGRAM (EEG)

The EEG is a noninvasive procedure that records the electrical activity on the brain's surface, called brain waves. It records the brain's ability to conduct electrical current in a smooth and uninterrupted manner, and aids in the establishment of the existence and types of epilepsy. Epilepsy or seizure disorders are the result of interruption in the electrical conduction (circuit) on the brain's surface, which may result from increased intracranial pressure, the lack of adequate peripheral cerebral blood flow, space-occupying lesions, and/or scar tissue from previous injuries. An EEG is also one of the criteria used in establishing brain death. Ideally all medications such as anticonvulsants, sedatives, tranquilizers, and stimulants are withheld 48 hours prior to the test. Of course, if the possibility of seizure activity exists, the anticonvulsants are not withheld. The procedure does not require any special preparation or nursing precautions. After the procedure, the patient needs a shampoo to cleanse the electrode paste from the hair and scalp.

ECHOENCEPHALOGRAPHY

Another noninvasive procedure, echoencephalography utilizes sound transmission and is useful in the diagnosis of subdural hematomas and midline structural shifts. The sound waves are recorded electrically from reflecting surfaces such as the cranial vault and the cerebral midline structures. It is a safe and rapid radiological or ultrasound study requiring no special precautions or nursing preparation.

PNEUMOENCEPHALOGRAPHY

An invasive procedure, this technique involves the injection of air or oxygen into the subarachnoid space by the lumbar or cisternal puncture method. Radiographic films are made for visualization of the intracranial subarachnoid space and the ventricles of the brain. It may be done for either diagnostic or therapeutic purposes. The therapeutic application of this procedure is breaking up posttraumatic subarachnoid adhesions that may have been causing severe headaches. Pneumoencephalography is contraindicated if there is evidence of greatly increased intracranial pressure with signs of papilledema or if intratentorial or supratentorial lesions are suspected. If such lesions are suspected and there are no alternatives for correct diagnosis, then emergency equipment (a drill set for burr holes) and adequate personnel must be on hand to deal with an emergent situation of increased intracranial pressure and possible brain herniation. With the cisternal puncture approach, the nape of the patient's neck must be shaved; with lumbar puncture the patient is prepared as for a routine spinal tap. The patient is given a sedative the evening prior to the procedure. He should have nothing by mouth past midnight, and a preoperative medication is given thirty minutes prior to the procedure. The premedication is atropine (dosage depending on the patient's size and age), with or without codeine sulfate. Clothing and items of jewelry, dentures, glasses or contact lenses, and hair pins must be removed. The patient should void prior to leaving his clinical area, and a complete set of vital signs and neurological assessment should be done and recorded. After the procedure, vital signs and neurological assessment are recorded every fifteen minutes until the patient's condition is stable (usually four to twelve hours) unless otherwise ordered by the physician.

SPINAL TAP OR LUMBAR PUNCTURE

The most commonly performed neurological diagnostic study and the only one that may be performed by physicians other than neurological specialists, the spinal tap is invasive and may be either diagnostic or therapeutic in nature. (For full details on spinal tap and cerebrospinal fluid analysis, see Chapter 3.)

RADIOGRAPHIC STUDIES

Radiographic studies, which are noninvasive and include skull and spinal X-rays, are discussed in Chapters 8 and 9.

CEREBRAL ANGIOGRAPHY

An invasive procedure, cerebral angiography is only diagnostic in nature. The contrast media (usually radiopaque dye) is injected into the cerebral circulation via the carotid artery and is followed by radiographic tracing to evaluate the cerebrovascular blood flow within the intra- and extracranial vessels. Visualization of the cerebral circulation aids in locating the cerebral arteries and veins and in determining their size and efficiency. Visualization of tumors, abscesses, aneurysms, hematomas, cerebral bleeds, and ventricular distortions can also be obtained with cerebral angiography.

The patient is prepared in the same manner as any other preoperative patient (except that there is no surgical shave for the female patient—the male patient's face and anterior neck are shaved the morning of the procedure). The preoperative medication and the type of anesthesia used during the procedure largely depend on the patient's clinical condition. Recording of vital signs and neurological assessments—both before and after angiographic studies—is mandatory. They are recorded every fifteen minutes for four to twelve hours, then every four for the next twelve hours, unless otherwise ordered. Because of the introduction of a dye, precautions against allergic reactions must be taken. Severe vascular spasms may also result; therefore emergency equipment and appropriate personnel must be on hand to intervene. Patients with suspected or confirmed sensitivity to iodine and/or shellfish should not undergo this procedure. The puncture site on the neck is usually dressed with a pressure dressing and ice packs are applied to control local edema.

VENTRICULOGRAPHY

Ventriculography is an invasive diagnostic procedure in which air or oxygen is injected into the lateral ventricles via ventricular puncture through the occipital, posterior parietal, or frontal lobe. Its specific purposes are to establish patency (the efficiency of the circulating cerebrospinal fluid) of the cerebral ventricular system, to determine the location of tumors, and to detect other cerebral anomalies. It is contraindicated if the presence of increased intracranial pressure is suspected, or if the subarachnoid space is to be studied also. (The procedure does not aid in the evaluation of the subarachnoid space.)

The patient is prepared in the same manner as any other preoperative patient and, in addition, the patient's hair must be clipped and shampooed the evening before the procedure. If a craniotomy is to follow the ventriculography, the patient's entire head is shaved. (Samples of the hair should be saved, as the patient's family may wish to purchase him or her a wig.) The procedure and its preparation will have a tremendous psychological impact on the patient and his family, and the nurse must provide the necessary support and reassurance for them.

After the ventriculogram is completed, the vital signs are recorded and neurological assessments are made every fifteen minutes for four to twelve hours, then every one to two hours for twenty-four hours, unless the condition warrants more frequent monitoring or the physician orders otherwise. The head of the bed is elevated fifteen degrees, and an ice cap is applied to the head to control mild headaches. If the ice cap does not control the headache, mild analgesics may be given as ordered. Narcotics or heavy sedatives are not used, because they may mask neurological clinical symptoms. The nurse must be constantly on the alert for signs of increasing intracranial pressure, and the slightest change in the patient's condition must be reported immediately to the physician. If hemorrhage occurs, respiratory collapse will follow unless the underlying condition is corrected promptly.

MYELOGRAPHY

An invasive procedure, myelography involves the injection of a dye (pantopaque or amipaque) or air via a lumbar puncture approach to establish the presence and degree of spinal cord compression. The contrast medium aids in visualization of the spinal canal and the spinal subarachnoid space, thus tracing the circulation of the cerebrospinal fluid and confirming suspected spinal nerve root compression or intravertebral disc rupture. The intravertebral discs are little pillow-shaped fibrous rings with a pulpy center situated between the vertebrae that prevent the bony surfaces from grinding together. They also aid in the forward flexion of the spine.

In preparation for a myelogram, the patient must take nothing by mouth for at least four hours prior to the procedure. The male patient may have to be shaved in the lumbar area. Administration of a cleansing enema may also be necessary for lumbar area studies to exclude shadows from the intestinal contents on the radiographic films. If the dye is removed, the patient may be kept flat in bed for four hours and allowed up thereafter to assume his previous activities. If the dye is not removed, his head must be kept higher than his trunk to keep the contrast media from gravitating to the brain, where it will cause cerebral meningeal irritation. This meningeal irritation, which is expressed by severe headache, is referred to as a spinal or post-myelogram headache. If the patient has had an air myelogram, his head is to be kept lower than his trunk for forty-eight hours. After forty-eight hours the air should have been absorbed so that there is no danger of it traveling up into the cerebral subarachnoid space and ventricles. This decreases the possibility of increased intracranial pressure or air embolism. Vital signs and neurological assessment should be done every fifteen minutes times four, then every hour times four if the patient's condition is stable. If the patient's condition remains unstable, these nursing functions must be done every fifteen minutes until his condition stabilizes or his physician orders otherwise.

BRAIN SCANNING WITH RADIOISOTOPES

This technique is about 80 to 95 percent accurate in the detection of metastatic tumors, malignant gliomas, and meningiomas that are highly vascular and rapid growing. If the tumors are relatively slow growing and avascular, as in the case of astrocytomas, the accuracy of detection is markedly reduced. In these cases a combination of radioisotope brain scanning and cerebral angiography is employed to assure 100 percent accuracy in localization and identification of brain tumors. Brain scanning is also useful in the detection of blood clots, infection, cerebral blood flow or vascular insufficiency, and abnormalities capable of displacing normal brain tissue. The radioactive substance, usually technetium 99m, is given intravenously. The patient is taken to the nuclear medicine department and placed in contact with the radioactive sensing device. The sensing device, a small crystal, records the localized concentration of the radioactive substance and transmits this information onto film or paper for interpretation. The interpretation is based on the established normal/abnormal brain tissue concentration (uptake) ratio. As a rule, the healthy brain tissue concentration of the radioactive substance will be much less than that of the pathological brain tissue. No adverse reactions result from brain scanning; thus special nursing considerations or care prior to or after the procedure are not required.

COMPUTER-ASSISTED TOMOGRAPHY

The CAT scan may or may not be invasive, but a large percentage of them are performed as noninvasive procedures. If the invasive method is employed, the same precautions for allergic reactions must be taken as with any procedure in which dye injection is utilized. Several different types or models of CAT scanners are available and utilized today. The most popular model is the ACTA (the automated-computerized transverse axial) scanner, which may be used for head or total body scans and requires a five-minute interval for each view. The patient does not have to be repositioned during the procedure, since the computer within the scanner directs the X-ray beams onto the specific areas for which it has been preprogrammed. The first computer within the scanner assimilates the gathered data into a black and white picture, while the second computer analyzes this picture and produces a colored picture that reflects the density of tissue in relation to the entry of the X-ray beam. It then prints out this information on tape, projects the picture onto an oscilloscope or screen, provides Polaroid pictures, and produces a numerical printout of the findings. Although it sounds as if the patient is in danger of major radiation exposure, it actually utilizes very little radiation—no more than what is utilized during a skull series radiographic study. ACTA scanning can therefore be repeated safely several times to monitor the progression or resolution of a disease process. It is commonly used for diagnostic purposes in head trauma, cerebrovascular disturbances, detection of space-occuping lesions, and hydrocephalus or cerebroventricular distentions. There are some disadvantages to CAT scans: (a) the high acquisition cost of the equipment is reflected in the cost of the test to the patient, and (b) the patient must remain perfectly motionless during the entire procedure, which may take from thirty minutes to two hours. If he is unable to remain immobile, he must be very heavily sedated and personnel and equipment must be on hand to deal with any possible emergent situation resulting from sedation. Of course, if the patient is unconscious a qualified nurse must accompany him to the scanning facility and remain with him. With the noninvasive CAT scan there are no special pre- or post-procedural nursing functions. With invasive scanning, the same nursing functions are done as for cerebral angiography, discussed earlier.

CALORIC TEST FOR VESTIBULAR FUNCTION

The caloric test is performed with water of extreme temperatures. Iced and very warm (112°F) water is used to test the vestibular portion of the eighth cranial nerve and aid in the differential diagnosis of lesions in the brainstem or cerebellum. The patient should have nothing by mouth for six hours. He should be given a full explanation of the procedure and be checked for nystagmus and perforation of the tympanic membranes (eardrums) prior to the test. If nystagmus, dizziness, and nausea do not occur, the results are said to be negative to thermal stimulation, and no disturbance of vestibular function is present. The caloric test is contraindicated if the tympanic membranes are perforated, or if otitis media, or Meniere's syndrome, is present.

GLUCOSE TOLERANCE TEST

This test is employed to rule out hypoglycemia as the underlying cause of seizure disorder, and it is also useful in detection of pituitary disease. The patient is kept fasting for eight to twelve hours prior to the test. He is then given a prepared glucose solution by mouth, a fasting blood sugar sample is drawn at this time, and serial blood samples obtained at intervals are compared with the fasting sample. After ingestion of the oral glucose solution, the blood sugar levels should rise within an hour and return to normal within two and a half hours. If the intravenous method is used, the blood sugar levels should rise within three minutes and return to normal within sixty to ninety minutes.

IODINE-STARCH SWEAT TEST

This noninvasive test is used in evaluating the sympathetic nervous system to detect the presence and extent of lesions within this system. The patient's body is painted with iodine, which is allowed to dry. It is then dusted with powdered starch. Skin surfaces are not allowed to touch. The patient is given pilocarpine subcutaneously to induce sweating. When sweating occurs, in about thirty minutes, the sweat dissolves the starch, which reacts with the iodine to produce dark purple areas over the healthy nerve tract. Where no reaction occurs, there is interruption to the sympathetic nervous system in that area. It will show up, for example, when a sympathectomy has been performed on a patient for pain control. *Caution:* This test is not to be performed on patients with known or suspected sensitivity to iodine.

All the previously mentioned tests except for spinal and skull X-rays require a written and signed consent from the patient or his legal representative prior to the procedure.

REFERENCES

Anthony-Parker, Catherine. *Textbook of Anatomy and Physiology.* 9th ed. Saint Louis: C. V. Mosby Company, 1975.

Arsenault, Linda. "Metastatic Cancer and the Nervous System." *Focus* 2, no. 6 (December 1984): 30–47.

Bates, Barbara. *A Guide to Physical Examination.* Philadelphia: J. B. Lippincott, 1974.

Bracke, Mary; Gill Taylor, Ann; and Kinney, Anna Belle. "External Drainage of Cerebrospinal Fluid." *American Journal of Nursing,* August 1978, p. 1355.

Braumlin, Dowd, and Jeri Lynn. Rook, Janice; and Sills, Grayce M. "Families in Crisis: The Impact of Trauma." *Critical Care Quarterly* 5, no. 3 (December 1982): 38–46.

Burrell-Owens, Lennett, and Burrell, Zeb L., Jr. *Intensive Nursing Care.* Saint Louis: C. V. Mosby Company, 1969.

Cannon, Maureen. "To Sharon with Love." *American Journal of Nursing,* April 1979, pp. 642–45.

Chusid, Joseph G. *Correlative Neuroanatomy and Functional Neurology.* 8th ed. Los Altos, CA: Lange Medical Publications, 1982.

Conway-Lang, Barbara. *Carini and Owens' Neurological and Neurosurgical Nursing.* 7th ed. Saint Louis: C. V. Mosby Company, 1978.

Dagi, T. Forcht. "Penetrating Missile Injuries of the Brain." *Critical Care Quarterly* 6, no. 1 (June 1983).

Davis-Sharts, Jean. "Mechanisms and Manifestations of Fever." *American Journal of Nursing,* November 1978, p. 1874.

Dorland, William Alexander. *Dorland's Illustrated Medical Dictionary.* 26th ed. Philadelphia: W. B. Saunders, 1981.

Dracup, Kathleen, and Weinberg, Sulvan Lee, eds. "Conference on Oxygen Therapy." *Heart and Lung* 13, no. 5 (1984): 550.

Edwards Smith, Alisa, and Nunn, Catherine K. "The Phrenic Nerve Stimulator." *Critical Care Nurse,* May/June 1982, pp. 78–81.

Frey, Charles. *Initial Management of the Trauma Patient.* Philadelphia: Lea & Febiger, 1976.

Hawken, Margarethe, and Ozura, Judith. "Practical Aspects of Anticonvulsant Therapy." *American Journal of Nursing*, June 1979, pp. 1062–68.

Hill, Martha. "Helping the Hypertensive Patient Control Sodium Intake." *American Journal of Nursing*, May 1979, pp. 906–9.

Jackson, Ludder Pat. "Ventriculo-Peritoneal Shunts." *American Journal of Nursing*, June 1980, pp. 1104–9.

Johnson, Joyce H., and Cryan, Maura. "Homonymous Hemianopsia: Assessment and Nursing Management." *American Journal of Nursing*, December 1979, pp. 2131–34.

Jones, Cathy. "Glasgow Coma Scale." *American Journal of Nursing*, September 1979, pp. 1551–53.

Kinney, Marguerite. "The Scientific Basis for Critical Care Nursing Practice: 1972 to 1982." *Heart and Lung* 13, no. 2 (March 1984): 116–21.

Kolthoff, Norma Jane. *Textbook of Anatomy and Physiology*. Saint Louis: C. V. Mosby Company, 1975.

Marcinek, Margaret. "What Hypertension Does to the Body." *American Journal of Nursing*, May 1980, pp. 928–37.

McCormick, Glenn P., and Williams, Margaret. "Stroke: The Double Crisis." *American Journal of Nursing*, August 1979, p. 1410.

Moser, Marvin. "How Hypertension Therapy Works." *American Journal of Nursing*, May 1980, pp. 937–41.

Norman, Susan. "Diagnostic Categories for the Patient with a Right Hemisphere Lesion." *American Journal of Nursing*, December 1979, pp. 2126–30.

Norman, Susan, and Baratz, Robin. "Understanding Aphasia." *American Journal of Nursing*, December 1979, pp. 2135–38.

Smith, Dorothy W., and Gipps, Claudia D. *Care of the Adult Patient: Medical-Surgical Nursing*. 2nd ed. Philadelphia: J. B. Lippincott, 1966.

Stipe, Jean; White, Dorothy; and Van Arsdale, Eleanor. "Huntington's Disease." *American Journal of Nursing*, August 1979, pp. 1428–33.

Sullivan, Maureen, and Jackson, Bettie S. "Tetanus—A Case Presentation." *Focus* 11, no. 3 (June 1984): 39–46.

Urosevich, Patricia, ed. *Coping with Neurologic Disorders*, Intermed. Philadelphia: Springhouse Publishing, Nursing Photobook 1982.

Vanden Zander, James W. *Social Psychology*. New York: Random House, 1977.

Wade, Jacqueline F. *Respiratory Nursing Care*. 2nd ed. Saint Louis: C. V. Mosby Company, 1977.

Wallhagen, Margaret I. "The Split Brain: Implication for Care and Rehabilitation." *American Journal of Nursing*, December 1979, pp. 2118–25.

Walt, Alexander J., and Wilson, Robert F. *Management of Trauma: Pitfalls and Practice*. Philadelphia: Lea & Febiger, 1975.

Wink, Diane. "Bacterial Meningitis in Children." *American Journal of Nursing*, April 1984, pp. 456–60.

GLOSSARY OF TERMS

ACIDOSIS: A condition of excessive hydrogen ion concentration in body fluids with serum pH less than 7.35.

ADAMS-STOKES SYNDROME: A syndrome of unconsciousness or convulsions resulting from inadequate cerebral blood flow associated with a high degree of heart block or transition from one rhythm to another, as with the onset of ventricular tachycardia.

ADRENERGIC CRISIS: A condition of extreme overactivity of that portion of the sympathetic nervous system mediated by epinephrine, producing epinephrine intoxication. Symptoms include hypertension, tachycardia and other arrhythmias, dry mouth, decreased intestinal motility, dilated pupils, anxiety, and psychotic behavior.

AGNOSIA: A disruption in the ability of the specific cerebral cortical area to effect sensory integration through the special senses—that is, vision, hearing, touch, and identification of the relationships of body parts.

ANAPHYLAXIS: An extreme sensitivity reaction characterized by shock and marked increase in capillary permeability producing soft-tissue edema; induced by external factors such as drug or food allergies, incompatible blood, insect bites, etc. This condition may be fatal if left untreated.

ANASARCA: A condition with generalized, massive edema involving the entire body. It may be both internal and external.

ANEURYSM: A sac-like bulging of a vessel wall, either weakened by disease or deriving from an abnormality at birth.

ANOXIA: Literally "without oxygen"; a condition of inadequate blood supply or inadequate oxygen content of the blood, resulting in tissue injury or death.

ANTICHOLINERGIC AGENT: A drug or chemical that blocks the transmission of impulses across the parasympathetic ganglia or blocks the effect of acetylcholine; antivagal in effect. Atropine is such an agent.

APHASIA: Inability to transmit, receive, or respond to ideas by language in any of its forms—speaking, reading, or writing. There are different types of aphasia: (a) expressive aphasia—inability to express one's wishes clearly in any of the above forms of communication; (b) receptive aphasia—inability to understand or comprehend components of the communication skills; (c) acute global aphasia—total inability to communicate, even with body language (by shrug, facial grimace, etc.). Information may be received and correctly interpreted, however. This state may sometimes be confused with coma.

APNEA: The cessation of breathing; it may be intermittent or permanent.

APRAXIA: A condition in which the individual cannot perform motor functions in response to specific directions, although there is no known motor impairment or diminished strength.

AREFLEXIA: The absence of reflex action (involuntary or automatic movement) with stimulation such as the knee jerk when the semiflexed knee is tapped with the percussion hammer.

ARGYLL ROBERTSON PUPIL: A condition in which the affected pupil is miotic, able to respond to near and far vision or accommodating, but does not respond to light.

ARRHYTHMIA: Without rhythm—out of time or sequence—such as an irregular heart beat.

ASCULTATION: The act of listening for sounds within the body, especially the lungs, heart, abdomen, and the blood vessels.

ASYNERGIA: Lack of sequential muscular contractions resulting in uncoordinated movements.

ATAXIC BREATHING: A respiratory pattern lacking rhythmic inhalation and exhalation. The patient is unable consciously to change this respiratory pattern even when asked to do so.

BABINSKI'S SIGN: Elicited by stroking the sole of the foot. The normal response is plantar flexion (forward flexion) of the great toe. If it is abnormal and dorsal flexion (curling under) of the great toe occurs, pyramidal tract involvement is suspected.

BETZ'S CELLS: The large ganglion (pyramidal) cells forming one of the layers of the motor area of the gray matter in the brain.

BIFURCATION: To divide into two branches.

BILIRUBINEMIA: An excessive amount of broken-down red blood cells within the body. The liberated heme (insoluble iron) portion of the hemoglobin gives the jaundice (yellow) appearance to the skin.

BIOT'S RESPIRATION: An irregular respiratory pattern of both rate and tidal volume (the amount of air inhaled with each breath), which is associated with central nervous system disturbances.

BRADYCARDIA: A slow pulse; a heart rate below sixty beats per minute.

BROWN-SÉQUARD SYNDROME: Results from damage to one half (vertically) of the spinal cord, resulting in paralysis and loss of discriminatory and joint sensation of the affected side, and loss of pain and temperature sensation on the opposite side of the body.

BRUDZINSKI'S SIGN: A sign of meningeal irritation. It is said to be positive or present if the patient cannot tolerate forward flexion of his neck onto his chest, due to severe pain, while lying in the recumbent position (flat on his back).

CAROTID ARTERY: The principle artery supplying blood to the head and neck, arising from the aortic arch on the left and the innominate artery on the right as they leave the heart.

CAROTID SINUS (BODIES): A collection of sensory cells near the bifurcation of the carotid artery that are highly sensitive to pressure and to the carbon dioxide concentration in the blood. These carotid bodies aid in the reflex control of the heart rate, the blood pressure, and the respiration.

CEPHALAD/CAUDAD: Upward toward the head/downward toward the feet.

CHEMORECEPTORS: Nerve cells that are sensitive to concentrations of certain chemicals.

CHEYNE-STOKES RESPIRATION: A cyclic-type respiratory pattern characterized by a period of apnea, followed by an increase in rate and depth of respiration until another period of apnea occurs. A common cause is acidosis affecting the respiratory center of the brain.

CHOLINERGIC: Stimulated, activated, or transmitted by choline; a term applied to nerve fibers that liberate choline (acetylcholine), a hormone, at a synaptic cleft to aid the conduction of a nerve impulse.

CLONUS: Repetitive, regular, rapid contractions of a muscle group once it has been stimulated, usually indicative of central nervous system disease and affecting the arms and legs.

COMA: An unconscious state during which there is no response to stimuli. This term should be applied only to deep comatose states. Since there are varying comatose states, one should specify and record the degree from light to deep, the type of stimuli used, and the elicited response.

CONCUSSION: Compression of the brain due to a blow to the head briefly suppressing the arousal system, with momentary loss of consciousness but without structural damage.

CONTRALATERAL: The opposite side.

CORTICAL: Referring to the cortex, the superficial layer of the brain, kidney, or adrenal glands.

CREMASTARIC REFLEX: The reflex reaction of the muscle fibers in the testis and spermatic cords resulting in penile erection. The absence of this reflex indicates damage to the first lumbar nerve segment. Yet, penile erection is seen sometimes with high thoracic and cervical spinal cord injuries in the immediate and acute post-traumatic phase.

CYANOSIS: A bluish color of the skin and mucous membranes resulting from an excessive amount of reduced (oxygen-free) hemoglobin in the blood stream.

DECEREBRATE POSTURING: The position of the prone patient in rigid extension with arms internally rotated at the shoulders, extended at the elbows, and pronated; wrists in rigid extension with fingers flexed at the second joints; legs extended at the hips and knees, with the ankles and toes flexed. An indication of lesions in the upper part of the brainstem.

DEMYELINATION: Destruction of the myelin sheath, one of the two coverings of the nerve fiber; seen in degenerative nerve diseases such as amyothrophic lateral sclerosis (Lou Gherig's disease) and multiple sclerosis.

DERMATOME: An area of skin supplied with afferent nerve fibers by a single posterior spinal nerve root. Also called dermatomic area.

DEXAMETHASONE: A glucocorticoid used as a dehydrator in cerebral edema (and spinal cord edema, at times). Other dehydrators used in cerebral edema are Mannitol, Urevert, magnesium sulfate, Lasix, and Edecrin.

DIAPHORESIS: Profuse perspiration (sweating), occurring naturally or induced by drugs, as in the Iodine-Starch Sweat test.

DIPLOPIA: Double vision, seeing two images while looking at one object.

DOLL'S EYES MANEUVER: Rapid head turning from side to side resulting in conjugate deviation of the eye movements in the direction away from the head movement. Indicative of lesion in the diencephalon.

DORSIFLEXION: Contraction (bending) toward the back.

ECLAMPSIA: A condition that occurs in pregnant women with hypertension, edema, and/or proteinuria (protein in the urine); symptoms are headaches, visual disturbances, and sometimes convulsions and coma. This condition may also be seen in patients with kidney failure due to uremia—an accumulation of toxic wastes in the blood, which are normally filtered out by the kidney and eliminated through the urine.

EDEMA: A collection of abnormal amounts of fluid in the interstitial spaces (the tissue between the cells).

ELECTROLYTE: A chemical that, when dissolved, dissociates into electrically charged particles; for example, Na^+, K^+, and Cl^-. It is capable of conducting an electrical current.

ENCEPHALITIS: Inflammation of the brain, usually viral in origin.

ENCEPHALOPATHY: A condition of abnormal brain function without pathological abnormalities, as from toxins or edema.

ENDARTERECTOMY: The surgical removal of material from the intima of an artery by the stripping away of the endothelial lining and adherent material; for example, carotid endarterectomy.

ENDOGENOUS: Originating from within.

EPIDURAL: Over the dura.

EPILEPSY: A group of conditions resulting in ectopic foci of cerebral cortical activity, producing episodic abnormalities of function, such as convulsions.

EXOGENOUS: Originating from without.

FIBRILLATION: Rapid muscular twitching.

FIBRINOLYTIC: An agent capable of dissolving fibrin, an insoluble protein, which plays a role in blood clot formation. Amicar (aminocaproic acid) is such an agent.

FLACCID: Without tone.

FOCUS: A specific location.

GLIAL CELLS: One of the two types of nerve cells that make up the nervous system. There are three types of glial cells: astrocyte, microglial, and oligodendroglial cells—they connect, support, and nourish the neurons.

GLUCOSURIA: Sugar in the urine. It is an abnormal condition, as urine should not contain sugar.

Glossary of Terms

GRAND MAL EPILEPSY: A generalized convulsive seizure that may be accompanied by tongue biting and loss of sphincter control.

HEMIANESTHESIA: Loss of sensation in one side (half) of the body.

HEMIPARESIS: Muscular weakness in one half of the body or body parts.

HEMIPLEGIA: Paralysis affecting one side of the body involving both the upper and lower limb, and may include the face on the affected side.

HOMOLATERAL: Same side (of the body). Opposite of contralateral.

HYDROCEPHALUS: A condition of increased cerebrospinal fluid within the cranium.

HYPERCARBIA: Also known as hypercapnia, a condition in which there is an excessive amount of carbon dioxide present in the blood—usually resulting from poor ventilation.

HYPERKINESIA: Excessive muscular activity.

HYPERPNEA: An abnormal increase of respiration both in depth and rate.

HYPERPYREXIA: An abnormally elevated body temperature (usually a temperature above 103°F).

HYPERTENSIVE ENCEPHALOPATHY: Vascular changes within the brain resulting from sustained and prolonged high blood pressure.

HYPOTHALAMUS: The highest center in the brainstem having to do with autonomic functions.

HYPOTONIA: A condition of diminished tone of the skeletal muscle with loss of resistance of muscles to passive stretching (the muscles involved are floppy and the patient cannot exert any pressure with them).

HYPOVOLEMIA: An abnormal decrease in circulating fluid (plasma) in the body.

ICTAL: Convulsive or seizuring state.

ISCHEMIA: Temporary anemia (stoppage of blood supply) of a part due to inadequate blood flow.

JACKSONIAN EPILEPSY: A specific type of convulsion that begins as a repetitive contraction of a single muscle group and then spreads first cephalad (toward the head), then caudad (toward the lower body).

KERNIG'S SIGN: A sign of meningeal irritation: the painful inability to extend the leg when the thigh is flexed on the abdomen.

Glossary of Terms

KETOACIDOSIS: An excessive accumulation of electronegative elements, in this case hydrogen ions, resulting from ketone (protein) bodies in the body tissues and fluids due to the body's inability to utilize protein. Seen in diabetic ketoacidosis with insufficient insulin to help utilize the injested protein.

KUSSMAUL RESPIRATION: A specific type of respiration characterized by rapid, deep, unlabored, forceful respiratory effort. Commonly seen in acidotic states.

LABILE: Subject to sudden variations; for example, labile emotional outbursts of post-CVA.

NUCHAL: Pertaining to the neck.

OLIGURIA: Diminished urinary output, although the fluid intake may be the same or increased.

OPISTHOTONOUS: The severe dorsiflexion (arching) of the spine and neck; a sign of meningeal irritation.

OTITIS MEDIA: An acute inflammation due to infection in the middle ear. The symptoms include pain in the ear, headache, swelling, heat, redness, and diminished hearing in the affected ear.

PALSY: Interference with normal function of nerve conductions; for example, in Bell's Palsy.

PAPILLEDEMA: Swelling of the optic disc, or nerve head, produced by interference with venous draining through the retinal vein; usually a result of increased intracranial pressure (ICP).

PARASYMPATHETIC NERVOUS SYSTEM: The portion of the autonomic nervous system consisting of ganglia having their origin in the cervical and caudal autonomic ganglia mediated by acetylcholine (cholinergic) and generally balancing and opposing the sympathetic nervous system.

PARAPLEGIA: The loss of power, sensation, and reflexes of the lower extremities, with loss of bladder and bowel control, usually resulting from a spinal cord injury.

PARESIS: A generalized muscular weakness, also known as partial or incomplete paralysis.

PATELLAR REFLEX: A deep tendon reflex, a contraction of the quadriceps femoris elicited by sharply striking the relaxed patellar tendon.

PERIPHERAL: On the surface.

PETECHIAE: A group of pinpoint, nonraised, perfectly round, purplish-red spots caused by intradermal (under the skin) or submucous hemorrhage (bleeding).

PETIT MAL EPILEPSY: Characterized by momentary loss of awareness and contraction of a muscle or small muscle group. There are no preceding warnings or aftereffects; a momentary vacant stare may be noticeable.

PLEXUS: A fine network of muscles or nerve fibers.

POLIOMYELITIS: An inflammatory process involving the anterior horn cells of the spinal cord, caused by a specific virus.

PSEUDOBULBAR PALSY: Spastic paralysis or weakness of the muscles innervated by the cranial nerves, such as the muscles of the face, pharynx, and tongue, resulting from bilateral lesions of the corticospinal tract.

PSYCHOMOTOR EPILEPSY: Characterized by loss of awareness, although performance of simple motor action is continued.

QUADRIPLEGIA: The sudden and complete loss of sensory and motor function resulting in paralysis of all four limbs.

RUBOR: Redness, one of the four cardinal signs of inflammation; the other three are calor (heat), dolor (pain), and edema (swelling).

SEPTICEMIA: Also known as blood poisoning, a systemic disease associated with the presence and persistence of pathogenic (capable of producing illness) microorganisms or their toxins in the blood stream.

SPASTIC: Having exaggerated muscle tone resulting from nerve disorder.

STUPOR: Unconsciousness during which motor response is elicited only by deep, painful stimuli application.

SUBLUXATION: Incomplete dislocation.

SWAN-GANZ LINE: A triple lumen catheter used as an aid in the correct fluid management of the critically ill patient by monitoring his cardiac output (the heart's efficiency and the circulating blood volume within the body).

SYMPATHETIC NERVOUS SYSTEM: The portion of the autonomic nervous system whose impulses are mediated by epinephrine, normally opposing and balancing the parasympathetic activity.

TACHYCARDIA: A rapid pulse—a heart rate over 100 beats per minute.

TABES DORSALIS: The tertiary (late or end stage) form of syphillis with degeneration of the dorsal columns of the spinal cord and of the sensory nerve roots, due to infection of the central nervous system with Treponema pallidum (the organism that causes syphillis). The symptoms include loss of sensory and motor coordination, loss of reflexes, trophic (wasting away) changes in muscles and joints, incontinence or retention of urine, and failure of sexual drive. The disease is slow but progressive and occurs mostly after middle age.

TREMULOUS: With tremors, shaking.

TREPHINE: To open the skull by drilling.

TURBID: Cloudy.

TURGOR: The usual elastic consistency of the healthy living tissue or skin. The loss of skin or tissue turgor results from hypovolemia or severe dehydration.

UREMIA: An excessive accumulation of urea and other byproducts of protein metabolism in the blood resulting from inadequate nephron (functional filtering unit of the kidney) function. The clinical symptoms of uremia include nausea, convulsions (seizures) or coma, and an azotemic breath (smelling like urine).

VENTRICLE: Fluid-filled cavities in the brain.

WATERHOUSE-FRIDERICHSEN SYNDROME: An acute catastrophic adrenocortical insufficiency occurring most commonly as a complication of adrenal hemorrhage in meningococcic meningitis.

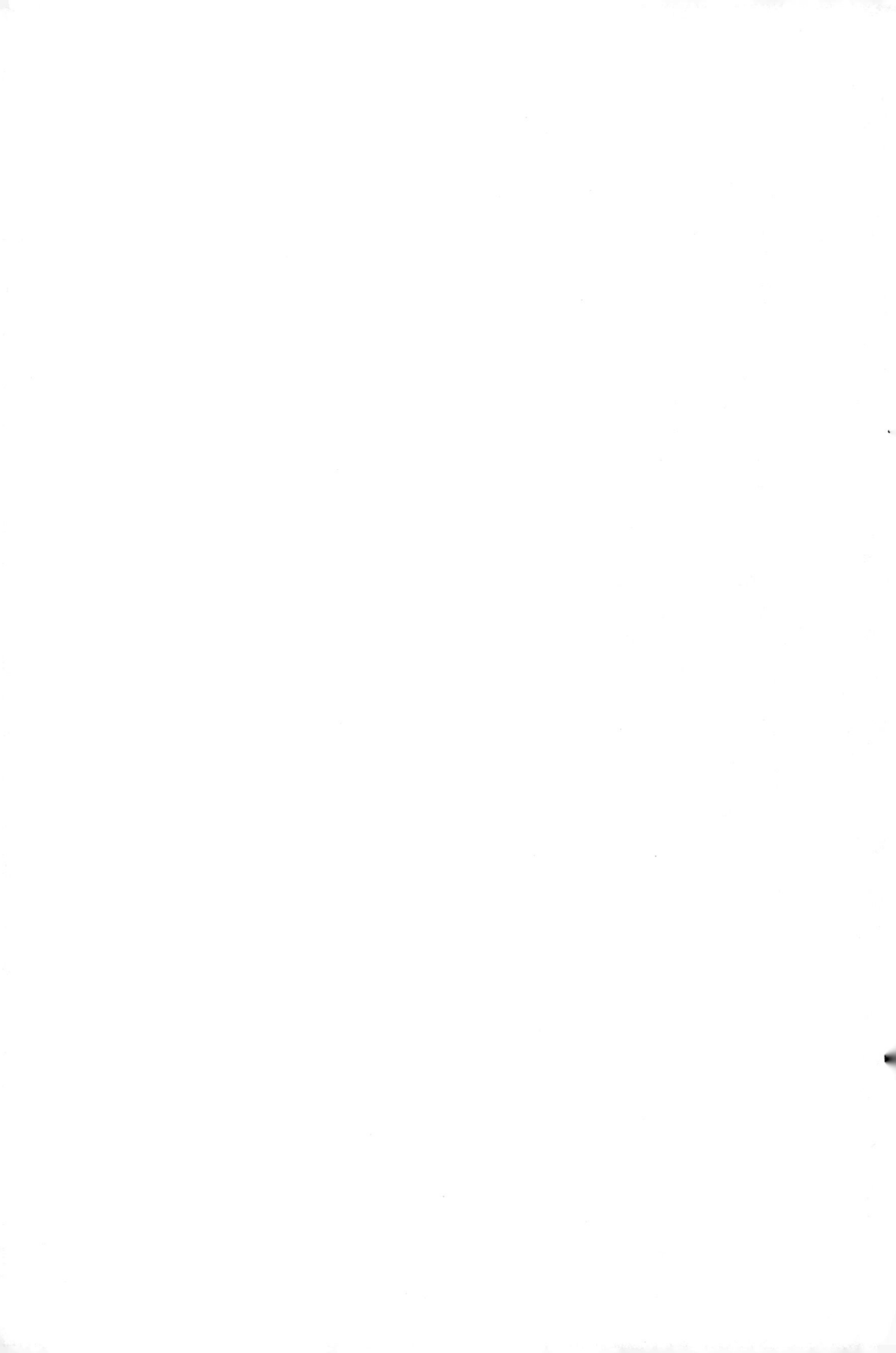

APPENDICES

MAJOR NEUROLOGICAL DRUGS
MOST COMMONLY USED IN THE MANAGEMENT OF THE NEUROLOGICAL AND NEUROTRAUMA PATIENT

Although a list of drugs available for use in the management of the neurological and neurotrauma patient would be nearly endless, a relatively small number are most frequently used. Their descriptions follow.

AMICAR (aminocaproic acid): A synthetic antifibrinolytic agent useful for stopping bleeding in medical and surgical conditions marked by hypofibriogenic hemorrhaging. It also can be used as antidote in overdosage of thrombotic (clot-disolving) agents, and may be given orally or intravenously.
Dosage: 5 gm oral or by slow IV, as a loading dose, then 1 gm every hour thereafter for two to three days.
Caution: Prolonged use of Amicar may induce blood clot formation; therefore, daily PPT (partial prothrombin time), PT (prothrombin time), and the Lee White clotting time tests are mandatory.

AMYTAL (sodium amobarbital): A barbiturate of intermediate duration. Its sedative effect is almost instantaneous when given intravenously, and it generally lasts 3 to 6 hours. It is given to control seizures in patients with status epilepticus when phenobarbital or Dilatin is ineffective.
Dosage: Repeated doses of 200 to 400 mg IV controls seizures very effectively.
Caution: As with any other sedative, respiratory embarrassment may occur and ventilatory assistance may become necessary. Administration of Amytal IV should not exceed 1 ml (200 mg) per minute or 1 gm/24 hours; it should be used within 30 minutes after reconstitution.

ASPIRIN (ASA): An analgesic and antipyretic (in neurotrauma nursing it is used for its antipyretic properties). As an antipyretic agent, it is given orally or rectally in suppository form, usually 10 grains every 3 to 4 hours.

Caution: Avoid giving it via naso-gastric tube if the patient is unconscious for a long time, as it may cause gastric irritation and bleeding. It may also interfere with blood clotting.

ATROPINE SULFATE: An anticholinergic, autonomic blocking agent. It blocks the action of acetylcholine from exerting its neurotransmitter action at the synaptic cleft. It is used chiefly as an antispasmodic to relax smooth muscles, as in gastric hypermotility and bronchial spasms, to reduce saliva production, and to increase the heart rate by blocking the vagus nerve. It is also used to dilate pupils for examination of the eyes, and as antidote for various toxic and anticholinesterase agents used in insecticides.

Dosage: 0.3 to 1.2 mg; may be given orally, intravenously, intramuscularly, or applied topically in drops or ointment forms.

Caution: Prolonged or overuse of atropine will result in tachycardia (too rapid heart rate) leading to coronary insufficiency and chest pain, constipation, urinary retention due to loss of bladder tone, blurred vision due to widely dilated pupils; is contraindicated in patients with glaucoma as it interferes with the drainage of aqueous humor (fluid in the eye ball).

BELLADONNA: Another autonomic blocking agent that acts the same as atropine, as atropine is a derivitive of belladonna (Atropa-belladonna).

Dosage: Depends on the preparation. It may range from belladonna extract 15 mg three to four times daily, to belladonna tincture 0.3 to 2.4 ml orally two to three times per day.

Caution: The same as for atropine.

CODEINE SULFATE: A narcotic alkaloid obtained from opium. It does not have the same respiratory depressant effect as morphine; however, it is used as an analgesic and, less frequently, as an antitussive, and is administered subcutaneously.

Dosage: 30 to 60 S. Q. every 3 to 4 hours, as needed for pain control (and at times for cough suppression).

Caution: It may cause chemical dependency in prolonged usage, and it does decrease gastric motility and may cause constipation.

DECADRON (dexamethason): A synthetic corticosteroid that causes less sodium and water retention than the natural glucocortical hormones and is about 35 times as potent. It is the most commonly used drug in management of cerebral edema, for its antiinflammatory properties, which prevent or reverse undesirable ultra-structural changes associated with cerebral edema. As the astrocyte (supporting structure for the neurons) swelling is reduced, intracranial pressure is decreased. The pooled fluid from the extracellular spaces is drawn back into the vascular system, with intracranial pressure decreasing as the tissue mass is reduced. It is also used in acute life-threatening emergencies.

Dosage: Loading dose 8 to 12 mg IV in severe cases, and 4 to 6 mg IV for maintenance dose every 6 hours thereafter. The dosage may vary, however, depending on the patient's clinical condition.

Caution: In case of prolonged use, dosage must by tapered prior to discontinuation. Peptic ulcer or systemic fungal infections may develop; meticulous IV site care is mandatory.

DILANTIN (diphenylhydantoin): An anticonvulsant; the most widely used drug for control of seizures.

Dosage: 0.3 to 0.9 gm daily for maintenance; however, the loading dose in status epilepticus is 1.2 to 1.5 gm IV given slow push *not to exceed 50 mg/1 minute*.

Caution: The patient must be on a cardiac monitor during administration of the drug, with resuscitation equipment available, as the drug may cause severe cardiac arrhythmias. Injection should be below the IV filter (it will otherwise occlude the filter), and it is not compatible with anything but saline; the line should therefore be flushed pre- and post-administration with saline.

KEFZOL, Ancef (sodium cephazoline): A semisynthetic cephalosporin, broad spectrum antibiotic for IV use. It can be used safely in patients who have a sensitivity to penicillin; in clinical applications it has been found to cross the blood-brain barrier fairly well.

Dosage: 0.5 to 1 gm IV every 4 to 6 hours. It may be given IM, but must be injected deep into the muscle.

Caution: After reconstitution, the drug is stable for 24 hours at room temperature and 96 hours under refrigeration. Cultures should be taken to establish the effectiveness of the drug. Renal toxicity may develop from prolonged use, and serial blood urea nitrogen studies should be done.

LASIX (furosemide): A high-potency, organic mercurial diuretic used in the management of both visable and nonvisable edema, as well as in some nonedematous conditions. It is used to treat congestive heart failure (lung congestion due to inefficient cardiac muscle tone); hepatic ascites (fluid collection in the abdomen due to liver failure); drug-induced edema, seen with cortisone therapy (corticosteriods cause fluid and sodium retention); edema of pregnancy resulting from hormonal imbalance; and in the control of hypertension. It may also be used in the reduction of intraocular pressure due to glaucoma, the reduction of increased intracranial pressure due to cerebral edema, in selected cases of epilepsy (seizure disorder), and occasionally in the treatment of poisoning to hasten renal (kidney) elimination of the toxic substance.

Dosage: Depending on the reason for use and the patient's clinical condition, it may range from 20 to 240 mg orally, intramuscularly or intravenously. In rare instances the intravenous dose may be as high as 1000 mg in one day.

Caution: It may cause severe electrolyte (mineral) disturbances, too-low blood pressure resulting in vascular collapse leading to convulsion (seizures) and coma. It is contraindicated in patients with severe kidney and liver impairment; patients on digitalis (a heart tonic) therapy, as it potentiates (strengthens) the action of digitalis; and insulin-dependent diabetic patients, as they may develop hyperglycemia (too-high blood sugar) and their insulin dosage must be adjusted to their needs. Tests to be done daily include serum electrolytes, blood urea nitrogen level (BUN), complete blood count (CBC) as it may produce leukopenia (reduction in white blood cell count) and thrombocytopenia (reduction in platelets—a factor in blood clotting). Accurate recording of fluid intake and urinary output is mandatory.

MANNITOL (Osmitrol): A sugar-derivative osmotic diuretic that increases renal blood flow, reduces vascular resistance and cerebral edema, resulting in decreased cerebrospinal fluid pressure.

Dosage: The average daily adult dose is 50 to 200 gm, but the dosage, concentration of the solution, and rate of administration will depend on the patient's clinical condition. It is given IV *only*. Administer below the IV filter site, since the molecular structure of Mannitol is too large to pass through. Commonly given in 12.5 gm 50 ml syringes and in 20 percent solution in 500 ml bottles.

NEMBUTAL (sodium pentobarbital): A sedative (barbiturate) that takes effect rapidly but lasts for a short time; only 3 to 4 hours. It is used to control convulsive seizures (if phenobarbital or Dilantin is ineffective), as a preanesthetic agent, and for the production of amnesia in obstetrics.

Dosage: To control seizures, 100 to 200 mg IV followed by 50 to 100 mg hourly, as needed. In severe head injuries, 50 to 100 mg hourly, IV, to suppress activity (which increases ICP).

Caution: Respiratory assistance and suctioning equipment must be readily available, and the patient must remain under constant nursing supervision. Therapy must be discontinued for 24 to 36 hours prior to an electroencephalogram (EEG) for the reading to be valid.

PARALDEHYDE (paral): A nonbarbiturate sedative used to control seizures, especially those induced by alcoholic withdrawal, since it is excreted through the lungs and not the liver.

Dosage: A 2 percent solution preparation may be administered by IV drip, 0.2 ml / kg body weight, or IM 5 to 7½ cc. It is available in 2, 5, and 10 ml ampules.

Caution: Do not expose to sunlight. Use glass IV bottles and syringes, because the drug will disintegrate plastic. It is not to be used in bronchopulmonary disease; if a cough develops, the rate of infusion must be decreased or the drug discontinued and another considered.

PENICILLIN: Any of a large group of natural or semisynthetic antibacterial antibotics derived directly or indirectly from strains of fungi. It has both bacteriocidal and bacteriostatic effects on many bacteria, especially gram-positive pathogens such as streptococci, staphylococci, pneumococci, and clostridia. It is also effective on some gram-negative pathogens such as gonococci, meningiococci, and the syphilis-causing Treponema pallidum spirochete organism. In addition to these it is effective in the treatment of some fungal infections.

Penicillin is available in a wide variety of strengths, and may be short- or long-acting. It may be given orally, intramuscularly, intravenously, intrathecally (into the spinal canal), and applied topically.

Dosage: Depending on the patient's diagnosis and clinical condition, it may range from Pen-Vee K 250 mg four times per day, to the long-acting penicillin-G in 1,200,000 units given intramuscularly as a single dose in the treatment of gonorrhea and syphilis.

Caution: Because of its overuse or misuse by the public, many people have developed hypersensitivity or allergy (drug intolerance) to penicillin. The allergic reaction may range from itching and hives to anaphylactic shock. The latter reaction is more common with a large, single-dose penicillin-G when given intramuscularly. A number of deaths have been reported from a single low dose oral penicillin such as Pen-Vee K, however.

PENTOTHAL (sodium thiopental): An ultra-short-acting barbiturate that produces basal, general anesthesia within seconds of administration and is therefore useful in overcoming acute, uncontrolled convulsions. It is rarely used in the emergency department or an intensive care unit unless a competent anesthetist is present, since paralysis of the medullary respiratory center may occur and endotracheal intubation must be performed.

Dosage: 50 to 75 mg IV (2 to 3 ml of the 2.5 percent solution) at 30- to 60-second intervals. Dosage should not exceed 1.5 to 3 gm, depending on the patient's body weight.

Caution: Ventilatory assistance and endotracheal intubation may be necessary. This drug should not be used on patients with history of respiratory and circulatory difficulties.

PHENOBARBITAL (sodium luminal): The single most-effective sedative used to control convulsive disorders, and the first-line drug in controlling status epilepticus. It does not take effect quickly, as it is slow to cross the blood-brain barrier, but its effects are of long duration. It produces sleep for at least six hours, followed by long periods of residual sedation. Its selective depressant action on motor neurons makes it especially useful in controlling epilepsy.

Dosage: 60 to 320 mg IV or IM to control status epilepticus and prevent convulsions following neurosurgery. Dosage is adjusted to the patient's needs.

Caution: Excretion is slow and the drug may accumulate, especially in patients with poor renal function. It is not recommended if daytime sedation is undesirable.

PITRESSIN (vasopressin): An antidiuretic hormone (ADH) formed by the neuron cells of the hypothalamic nuclei and stored in the posterior pituitary gland. Its main function is the control of water metabolism, and it is used in the treatment of diabetes insipidus. This disorder is accompanied by excessive sugar-free urinary output, with specific gravity of 1.001 or 1.000, and results in severe dehydration. The condition is common in patients with severe cerebral trauma and postoperative neurosurgery occurring after about three days, when the positive water balance phase has passed. The drug helps concentrate the urine and increases reabsorbtion of water from the renal tubules. Its release is determined by the osmolality of the plasma.

Dosage: 0.5 ml containing 10 units Pitressin, water base, IV for rapid response, and 10 units Tannate, in oil IM for slower response. It may be repeated every 6 hours if the urinary output is greater than 8 liters in 24 hours or exceeds 300 cc per hour for 3 consecutive hours.

Caution: Overdosage may result in water intoxication (volume overload), which in turn will cause a rise in BP and ICP. In case of overdose, Lasix, 20 to 40 mg IV, is given. Hourly urine tests are mandatory, and specific gravity along with serum osmolality tests should be done.

PROSTIGMIN (neostigmin): A cholinergic autonomic neuroeffector drug used in the diagnosis and treatment of myasthenia gravis to stimulate nerve impulse transmission and increase muscular contraction. It is given in small doses of 0.25 to 1 mg IM or SC, since large doses can lead to blockage of the nerve impulse transmission, resulting in muscular paralysis. In addition to the long-term treatment of myasthenia gravis and emergency treatment of myasthenia crisis, it has many other uses; for example, as a diagnostic aid in peripheral nerve injury, and for the reduction of intraocular pressure in wide-angle glaucoma.

Caution: The use of Prostigmin is to be avoided in patients with peptic ulcer and spastic or obstructive gastrointestinal disturbances, in patients with bronchial asthma, narrow-angle glaucoma, and acute renal failure, and in patients with cholinergic crisis.

TENSILON (edrophonium chloride): Another cholinergic drug used in the diagnosis of myasthenia gravis and the treatment of myasthenia crisis. It may also be used as an antidote in the overdosage of curare, a respiratory muscle-paralyzing agent used during administration of general anesthesia prior to endotracheal intubation. Curare is given to relax the throat and thereby minimize the soft tissue injury during endotracheal intubation.

Dosage: 5 to 20 mg per day. The initial test dose is 2 mg IV, however, and it is not the primary choice of drug in the long-term treatment of myasthenia gravis.

Caution: Same as for Prostigmin.

TAGAMET (cimetidine): An antagonist to histamine H_2 receptors that inhibits gastric acid secretion in response to the stimuli of stress. It is especially effective in prevention and treatment of gastric (stress) ulcers.

Dosage: 300 mg every 6 hours IV (partial fill), or orally four times daily.

Caution: May cause severe psychosis, which clears within 48 hours after withdrawal of treatment. Administration is not to exceed 2400 mg / 24 hours.

THORAZINE (chlorpromazine hydrochloride): A major tranquilizer or antipsychotic agent. Although the clinical indication for its use is to quiet the severely disturbed hyperactive psychotic patient, as in acute schizophrenic reaction or the manic (active) phase of manic depressive (quite-withdrawn) psychosis, it is often used to control major motor (grand mal) seizures. In addition, it may be used to control nausea or vomiting and to enhance the action of narcotics (pain medication). Thorazine can be given in large doses without the side effects of respiratory depression.

Dosage: 30 to 1200 mg per day depending on the severity of the patient's symptoms and his response to the drug. It is given orally or intramuscularly.

Caution: Reduced vasoconstriction results in low blood pressure especially upon standing (postural hypotension); blurred vision and photo (light) sensitivity may also occur. These must be taken into consideration during eye examination, and the patient should not be exposed to direct sun as he may sustain severe sunburn.

TYLENOL (acetaminophen): An antipyretic, mild analgesic with less antiinflammatory effect than aspirin. On the other hand, it has very few side effects, as it does not interfere with anticoagulants or blood clotting. If used orally, it does not cause gastric distress and is well tolerated by patients with aspirin sensitivity.

Dosage: 650 mg every 2 to 3 hours for temperature greater than 101° F. Given rectally, orally, or via nasogastric tube, 32 ml of the 120 mg. per 5 cc elixir.

UREVERT (urea USP, carbamide, ureaphil): An osmotic diuretic dissolved in invert sugar creating a hypertonic solution that is very effective in the reduction of cerebrospinal edema and increased intracranial pressure. It is widely used in patients with neurotrauma or post-craniotomy. It is also effective in control of vascular headache and projectile vomiting, which are common in head and spinal cord trauma patients or those with meningeal irritation. Urevert is also used to reduce intraocular pressure in glaucoma, prior to repair of detached retina, and in controlling oliguria in burned patients.

Dosage: 100 to 1,000 mg per kg body weight IV in a 30 percent solution per day.

Caution: Rapid administration may cause diabetes-like hyperglycemia, congestive heart failure, and soft tissue injury in case of extravasation (tissue sloughing will result).

VALIUM (diazepam): A tranquilizer-sedative that depresses the central nervous system. It is often used for rapid control of convulsions. *However, its use is not advisable in other than the control of seizures resulting from alcohol withdrawal and the control of muscle spasms in cerebral palsy.*

Dosage: 5 to 20 mg IV to achieve sedation.

Caution: Not to be used in patients with glaucoma, and careful consideration should be given to its use in conjunction with other barbiturates, narcotics, or tranquilizers, as it potentiates their effect. Give below the IV filter site, and keep in mind to pre- and post-flush with saline, as Valium is not compatible with anything else.

ABBREVIATIONS

ADH: Antidiuretic hormone. It is the body's water and electrolytes (minerals) regulatory hormone and is in part responsible for the body's fluid balance.

BUN: Blood urea nitrogen. One of the waste by-products of protein metabolism in the blood. The normal blood urea nitrogen level is 8 to 25 mg per deciliter or 2.9 to 8.9 milimoles per liter, expressed as 8–25 mg/dL or 2.9–8.9 mmol/L.

CNS: Central nervous system. It is one of the nine body systems, and its organs include the brain, spinal cord, nerves, and ganglia.

CPP: Cerebral perfusion pressure. It is the existing pressure difference between the arterial and venous pressure within the brain or cranium; the normal range is 50 to 90 mm Hg.

CVA: Cerebrovascular accident or "stroke." It is one of the two major bleeding disorders in the brain resulting from a ruptured (broken) or blocked blood vessel. It may be either arterial or venous.

GCS: Glasgow Coma Scale. A system for recording neurological assessment data. See Figure 5.2.

ICP: Intracranial pressure. It is the existing pressure within the cranium (head). The normal intracranial pressure is 0 to 15 mm Hg or 0 to 20 cm H_2O.

MAP: Mean arterial pressure. It is the existing blood pressure within the body at any given time, and the normal range is 120 mm Hg systolic over 80 mm Hg diastolic pressure.

RAS: Reticular activating system—the nuclei in the brainstem in reticular formation and tracts to and from it.

SAH: Subarachnoid hemorrhage. It is a major intracranial bleeding episode occurring in the subarachnoid (the middle layer of the brain's covering); the blood displaces the cerebrospinal fluid in the subarachnoid space, resulting in severe meningeal irritation.

TIA: Transiant ischemic attack. This condition results from temporary functional constriction or actual obstruction of a blood vessel within the brain, and the symptoms resemble a stroke.

INDEX

abdominal reflex, 33
abducens nerve, 41
acetylcholine, 11
acoustic nerve, 41–43
adrenergic nerve fibers, 35
afferent neurons, 5
alignment of spinal cord, 76
Amicar, 87
angiography, cerebral, 85, 86–87, 97–98
ankle jerk, 32
anoxia, 59
anterior horn neurons, 29
antibiotics, 90
aphasia, 16
arachnoid membrane, 12–14
Argyll Robertson pupil, 39
arterial blood gases (ABGs), 59
assimilation, 78–79
astrocytes, 5
autonomic nervous system, 34–36
axons, 8, 35

Babinski reflex, 32–33
balance, 41–42
basal ganglia, 14–15
basilar skull fracture, 19–20
Biot's respiration, 59
bipolar neurons, 5
bony mineralization of the spinal cord, 76
bradycardia, 59
brain, 12–20
brain scanning, 100–101

Brudzinski's sign, 89
bruits, 85

caloric test, 102
cartilage space of the spinal cord, 76
CAT scan, 85, 101–2
central cord syndrome, 72
central nervous system
    injuries to, 56–58
    lesions in, 17
    organs of, 12
    and unconsciousness, 57
cerebellum, 18–19
cerebral angiography, 85, 86–87, 97–98
cerebral contusion, 68
cerebral cortex, 14–16, 28
cerebral laceration, 68
cerebral perfusion pressure (CPP), 47
cerebral vascular accident (CVA), 30, 82–86
cerebrospinal fluid, 14, 85, 92
cerebrospinal fluid (CFS) pressure, 25–27
Cheyne-Stokes respiration, 59
cholinergic nerve fibers, 35
cholinesterase, 11
circulation, 78
cochlear branch of the acoustic nerve, 42–43
coma, 58, 84
communication, 4

concussion, 67–68
conduction, impulse, 10
contusion, cerebral, 68
convergence, 29
convulsions, 62–64
corneal reflex, 33
corticospinal tracts, 29–30, 31
cough reflex, 33
cranial nerves, 37–45
craniotomy, 69, 99
Crutchfield tongs, 77

decerebrate posturing, 50–51
decorticate posturing, 50
dendrites, 8
dermatome, 73
deviation of the eyes, 44
diabetes insipidus, 66–67
diagnostic studies, 95–103
diuretic therapy, 66
divergence of the eyes, 44
divergence principle, 28
doll's eyes phenomenon, 44–45
dual autonomic innervation, 35
dura mater, 12
dysconjungate gaze, 44

echoencephalography, 96
edema, 48, 66
education, patient, 94
efferent neurons, 5
electroencephalogram (EEG), 15, 85, 89, 95–96
elimination, 79
embolism, cerebral, 83–84
emotional needs, 67, 80–81
encephalitis, 88–89
epidural hematoma, 68
epidural probe, 51
epilepsy, 63–64, 95–96
equilibrium, 41–42
extrapyramidal tracts, 30–31
eyes, 39–40, 44–45, 62

facial nerve, 41
facilitatory tracts, 30–31
falx cerebelli, 12
falx cerebri, 12
family, 67, 81
filum terminale, 22
final common path, 29
flaccid paralysis, 73, 74
fluids, 66, 79
foramen magnum, 19
fundus, 39

gag reflex, 33
glossopharyngeal nerve, 43
glucose tolerance test, 102–3
grand mal seizure, 64

head injuries, 19–20, 56, 65–69
hearing, 42–43
hematoma, 68–69
hemispheres, 14
hemorrhage, 83–84, 86–87
hormones, 11
hypertension, 59, 82–83
hypoglossal nerve, 44
hypotension, 59
hypothalamus, 17
hypothermia, 60

impulse conduction, 10
incomplete transection of the spinal cord, 72–73
intracerebral hematoma, 69
intracranial hematoma, 68
intracranial pressure (ICP), 46–52, 58, 66
iodine-starch sweat test, 103

Jacksonian (focal) seizure, 64
junctions, neuromuscular, 11

Kernig's sign, 89
knee jerk reflex, 32

laceration, cerebral, 68
language, 16
lateral spinothalamic pathway, 28
lobes, 14, 16

mandibular branch of the trigeminal nerve, 40
maxillary branch of the trigeminal nerve, 40
mean arterial pressure (MAP), 47
medial lemniscal pathway, 28–29
medication, 79–80
medulla oblongata, 19–20
memory, 54–55
meninges, 12
meningitis, 89–90
microglia, 5
midbrain, 18
morale, 67, 80–81
motor integration, 55
motor neural pathways, 29–31
motor neurons, 5
multipolar neurons, 5
myasthenia gravis, 92–94
myelin sheath, 8
myelography, 99–100

nerves
  cell types, 4–11
  cranial, 37–45
  of the peripheral nervous system, 73
  spinal, 22–25
nervous system
  autonomic, 34–36
  cellular structure of, 4–11
  central, injuries to, 56–58
  central, lesions in, 17
  central, organs of, 12
  central, and unconsciousness, 57
  peripheral, 73
neural pathways, 10, 27–31

neurilemma, 8
neurofibrils, 8–10
neuroglia, 4–5
neurological deficit, 48, 53–56, 70–74
neuromuscular junctions, 11
neurons, 5–11, 29, 34–35
Nissl bodies, 10
nucleus cuneatus, 20
nucleus gracilis, 20
nutrition, 79
nystagmus, 44

oculomotor nerve, 39–40
olfactory nerve, 37
oligodendroglia, 5
olive, 20
ophthalmic branch of the trigeminal nerve, 40
optic nerve, 37–39
oral care, 41, 62
otitis media, 43

palatal reflex, 33
papilledema, 39
paralysis, 73, 74
parasympathetic nervous system, 34–35
paroxysmal atrial tachycardia, 43
partial transection of the spinal cord, 72–73
patellar reflex, 32
peduncles, cerebellar, 18
peripheral nervous system, 73
peripheral sensory neurons, 8
peripheral vision, 39
petit mal seizure, 64
pia mater, 12–14
pneumoencephalography, 96–97
pneumotaxi center, 18
poliomyelitis, 87
pons, 18
post-ganglionic neurons, 34–35

posturing, 50–51, 92
pre-ganglionic neurons, 34–35
progressive neurological deficit, 48
Prostigman, 94
protein, 10
psychological components, 67, 80–81
psychomotor seizure, 64
psychosomatic disorders, 36
pulse, 60
pupil, 39–40, 60
pyramidal tracts, 29–30, 31
pyramids, 20

radiographic studies, 75–76
radioisotopes, 100–101
receptors, 8, 10
reflex arcs, 10, 34
reflexes, 32–34
reflexive activity, 73, 74
regeneration, 8
respiration, 59
reticular activating system (RAS), 31–32
reticulospinal tract, 30
retina, 37–39
Rinne test, 42–43

Schwann's cells, 8
seizures, 63–64, 95–96
sensory integration, 54–55
sensory neural pathways, 27–29
sensory neurons, 5
shock, spinal, 73
single autonomic innervation, 35
skin care, 79
skull fractures, 19–20, 69
soft tissue of the spinal cord, 76–77
somatic effector pathways, 34–35
somnolence, 58
spastic paralysis, 73, 74

spatial compensatory mechanisms, 46–47
speech, 16
spinal accessory nerve, 43–44
spinal cord
  injuries to, 56
  injuries to, evaluation of, 74–77
  injuries to, management of, 77–81
  injuries to, types of, 70–74
  structure of, 21–27
spinal nerves, 22–25
spinal shock, 73
spinal tap, 25–27, 97
  and meningitis, 89
  and poliomyelitis, 87
  and strokes, 85
  and subarachnoid hemorrhage, 86
stimulus, 10
stress, 36
strokes, 30, 82–86
stupor, 58
subarachnoid (Richmond) screw, 51
subarachnoid hemorrhage, 86–87
subarachnoid space, 14
subdural hematoma, 68–69
subdural space, 14
suctioning, 19–20
surgery, 65, 77
swallowing reflex, 33
sympathetic nervous system, 34–35
synapse, 10–11

tachycardia, 43, 59
temperature, 60
Tensilon, 94
tentorium cerebelli, 12
tetanus, 90–91
thalamus, 17, 28

thrills, 85
thrombosis, cerebral, 83–84
thymus gland, 93
traction, 77
transtentorial herniation, 47–48
trigeminal nerve, 40–41
trochlear nerve, 40

unconsciousness, 57–62, 84
unipolar neurons, 5–8

vagus nerve, 43

vehicular collisions, 56
ventilation, 59, 78
ventral spinothalamic pathway, 28
ventriculography, 98
ventriculostomy, 51
vertebral column, 21, 70
vestibular branch of the acoustic
 nerve, 41–42, 102
visceral functions, 16, 34
vision, peripheral, 39
visitation, 80–81